Healthy Meal Prep

The Secret to Make Healthy Eating Easier than Ever Before with a Delicious, Easy and Time Saving 6 Week Meal Prep Plan to Start Your Journey

By Chloe Hargreaves

Table of Contents

Introduction 4

Chapter 1: Why meal Prep? 8

Chapter 2: Why Most People Fail At Healthy Eating 15

Chapter 3: How to change your displeasure into success in a healthy meal plan 23

Chapter 4: How to avoid making the same mistakes in a healthy diet plan 27

Chapter 5: Setting your personal goals 36

Chapter 6: The Meal Prep Fundamentals 48

Chapter 7: Tips To Make Meal Prep Easier And Faster 54

Chapter 8: Kitchen Tools We Need For Meal Prep 58

Chapter 9: How to go BPA free 68

Chapter 10: How to Store Different Types of Foods 74

Chapter 11: Food Hygiene Tips for Your Fridge 78

Chapter 12: Purchasing Exact Amounts of Food to Save Time and Money 84

Chapter 13: Vegan Cooking Tips and Tricks . 90

Chapter 14: Tips for Losing Weight on a Vegan Diet..95

Chapter 15: Make a Grocery List 100

Chapter 16: How to make boring food tasty with ingredients...117

Chapter 17: Instructions to Make Boring Food Taste Amazing 123

Chapter 18: Preventing Foodborne Illnesses 126

Chapter 19: Meal plan for 6 weeks 142

Chapter 21: Freezer Meals 189

Chapter 22: Shopping Lists 199

Introduction

With busy calendars going all out, keeping up a healthy diet can be challenging. Meal preparation is one approach to control your food intake for a stress-free, financially effective approach in accomplishing your summer diet objectives. Regardless of how far you take it, meal planning is designed to ensure you have sufficient energy to truly think about your food consumption and make meals you will enjoy and can take in different ways, shapes, and forms.

Meal planning allows you to eat the meals you love while pre-packaged portions ensure you don't enjoy. Having a group of customized meals on hand will enable you to control what you eat and help you remain on track with your diet objectives.

Basically, meal prep implies planning for meals. And while single-serve meals are the best method for meal prep, there are different ways to prepare meals depending on your calendar, tastes, and dietary needs.

Kinds of meal prep include:

- ➢ Full make-ahead meals: You cook a whole meal and store it in your fridge or freezer.
- ➢ Batch cooking or freezing: Make different meals, then divide and store them. This approach is ideal for recipes you can easily cook in huge amounts (like big pots of soup, rice, or mashed sweet potatoes).
- ➢ Meals for one: Prepare food and store it in single-serving containers. (Usually enough to last a couple of days.)
- ➢ Ingredient prep: For people who like to cook and serve food all on the double, just prep parts of recipes. Cut veggies, mix flavors, or marinade meat in advance to spare time when you're ready to cook.

If the health benefits alone have not persuaded you to think about meal planning, think about the financial gains. Having food prepared at home will enable you to set aside some money as it keeps you from eating out. In addition, meal planning gives you full oversight over ingredients, enabling you to specifically look for staple goods. With an appropriate plan, you can avoid making pointless food purchases, saving you money and reducing food waste.

Meal plan requires, well, planning! Plan ahead. Think about your financial plan, favorite foods and above all - think about your objectives. Come up with recipes that incorporate ingredients from every food group to guarantee balanced meals (including protein, starch, and vegetables). Then, make a basic supply list, outline portions, and begin cooking!

Learning how to meal prep will not only spare you time, but it also saves some money and reduces waste. And unlike ready meals, this approach gives you control over what goes in your food — ideal for anyone who wants to stay on track with their health objectives. ?

Chapter 1: Why meal Prep?

I am a big supporter of meal prep. You don't have to be a bodybuilder to participate, and it saves loads of time in the week when you generally have little to spare. I know it seems like a difficult task, but it's importance in achieving your goals really can't be underestimated. Knowing what to eat, how much to eat, when to eat, and then preparing your meals is one of the most important aspects of achieving a healthy, balanced diet.

The key to getting ahead with meal prep is to have a few staple foods that you can batch-cook and use in a number of different ways. If you really don't have the time, opt for tinned fish, salads, raw veggies (think carrot sticks, cucumber, avocado, tomatoes, capsicums), fruit and nuts, which take zero time to throw in a Tupperware.

Take that extra time to prepare for the week ahead and you'll be rewarded with:

You will avoid food waste

According to a survey conducted by the American Chemistry Council, the average household in the United States throws out $640 of food each year. More than 50 percent of households throw out food every single week. If you are concerned about food waste, then meal prepping will reduce the amount of excess food that sits in your refrigerator before ending up in the trash. When you know exactly what you're going to make, you can buy the right ingredients in the proper portions.

You can enjoy the freshest food in season.

When you shop mindfully with a focus on good taste and good health, you can enjoy local fresh fruit and vegetables and other seasonal goodies. Combine pumpkin into your fall meals and asparagus when spring rolls around to enjoy fresh food and flavors.

Better Nutrition

Having your meals on hand during the day means you don't have to go to the local cafe for food. This not only saves you time, but also improves your waistline. You have full control over the portions and ingredients.

Improved Metabolism

You'll be ready at snack time when hunger strikes with something nourishing, so you can feed your body regularly and keep your metabolism humming. Snacking regularly will stop your body from falling into a catabolic state, which results in the loss of lean body tissue (including muscle) and slowing down of your metabolic rate.

More Money
Another major advantage of planning and prepping your meals is saving money. Skip the $15 a day you spend on a salad covered in croutons and unknown dressings (yuk), and you'll pocket $75 a week. That's enough for a new gym top AND an extra workout class!

Reduced grocery store trips.
If your weekly menu is planned ahead of time, you can do your best to buy everything for the week in one trip (unless you somehow still forget things like me).

Reduces wandering at the grocery store.
I'm a wanderer. Even when I have a list, I sometimes just want to search for sales or find yummy new items. But too much wandering wastes time.

Know what needs to be prepped (and prep it).
You know the menu, so you know what needs to be prepped. For example, we put diced onion in almost everything. So instead of dicing a little bit for every other meal, we dice the whole thing at once. You might not think about it, but that saves you the time you would use washing and drying your knife and cutting board for the next 3 or 4 times you need diced onions. And, if I have time now, I'll dice the other veggies for later too. Save time when you can by doing things you might not consider huge time savers. But they work.

Planned leftovers.
What can I say? I love leftovers. I'll stop trying to make "planned-overs" happen if you guys just admit leftovers save time. Isn't it obvious?

Eating the right amount.
I've sort of always done this thing where if it's on my plate, I'm eating it. And sometimes if you're feeling excessively hungry, way too happy to be eating, or just using a differently sized spoon, you can get totally varying/random portion sizes on the plate.

Planning and pre-portioning your food can ensure your hard work makes it to all 4 portions, instead of only 2.75 (oops!).

You will save calories.
When you can plan healthy meals ahead of time, you will be far less tempted to head to the fast-food drive-through, the office vending machine, or your junk food drawer. Likewise, having healthy meals on the go means you can enjoy good food at your convenience. Meal prepping also creates instant portion control. When your meals are pre-portioned, you will be less likely to overindulge or keep eating even after you are full.

Staying accountable to the past you.
If you already made the food and pre-portioned it into perfect bowls with future you in mind, you're really kicking the past you in the butt if you don't eat it. Planning and prepping your meals provides a little more incentive to eat the healthy things you've already planned out and cooked.

You save will power for other important life tasks.
Researchers in behavioral psychology have learned that will power can run out. Once you use it up, it is gone for the day. This may explain the term yo-yo dieting. By the end of the day, your decision-making abilities have been exhausted, which is precisely why ice cream shops and fast food restaurants stay open late.

More control over your choices.
If you know you have a dinner event or work lunch out, you can simply plan around it. Eat lighter for the rest of the day so you can indulge later. Or don't indulge, just plan. Either way, planning out your choices ahead of time means you are more likely to stick with the healthy choices you already made.

It is healthy and portion-controlled.
When you prepare your meals in your kitchen, you are not adding excess sodium, fat or sugar, like restaurants do. When the food is divided up and stored in containers, it is portioned out into the right amount of protein, carbohydrates, and fats. Dr. Brian Wansink,

Ph.D. and author of Mindless Eating has performed numerous studies on portion control. We will continue to eat if the food is in front of us, and can end up eating excessive amounts of calories. If we consume food out of a pre-portioned container, then once it is empty, we are done and do not stuff ourselves sick.

Chapter 2: Why Most People Fail At Healthy Eating

I grew up eating plenty of bacon, hotdogs, and unhealthy food and drank my espresso with no less than two teaspoons of sugar. White bread and butter were constants in my life, too. Actually, I adamantly believed that it would be difficult for me to ignore those foods from my diet without pain and sacrifice. Thinking back now, I understand how wrong I was.

A large number of us have tried to eat healthier and improve our diets at one time in our lives. However, the vast majority of us fail in our efforts and return to our old ways. We miss the foods we are used to eating and give up after a couple of days. The desires and 'sacrifice' we experience appear to be too overwhelming to survive, so we quit, wave the notorious white banner, and return to our old dietary patterns.

Unfortunately, many people who want to change their diet and eat healthier find it challenging and blame their inability to do so on their absence of self-control and resolve. But, in my experience, there are several reasons why many fall short.

People Are Too Hard On Themselves
One of the most widely recognized reasons why many people fail to stick to a diet is because they are too hard on themselves. If you were used to eating fast food and sugary things and without warning, change to a diet based exclusively on fruits or vegetables, your body will find it incredibly difficult to adjust. These sudden changes usually don't end up well – you can ruin yourself from time to time all through the diet, as long as you don't binge on desserts. If your body goes into starvation mode, it is almost impossible for you to fight the temptation to eat the food you were used to. Diets must be achieved slowly but surely, not suddenly.

They Do Not Track Progress
This is another one of the reasons people fail to maintain a healthy diet. If you don't weigh in advance, you are unlikely to know how much weight you have lost and this can be very frustrating to most of us. In the end, you can't track your progress (or tell whether there is any progress whatsoever) if you don't follow your weight loss efforts.

They Focus Solely On the Diet
In most cases, the diet alone won't help you to get thinner – or, better stated, it won't help you lose a lot of weight. If you have high weight loss objectives, the diet you pursue must be

accompanied by the right lifestyle changes. Many people neglect to maintain their diet because they don't pair it with two basic elements for effective weight loss: quality night's rest and normal physical activities.

Lack of Moral Support from Friends or Family

Moral support is basic for those who are attempting to shed pounds, as this is a real and difficult plan that requires plenty of confidence and resolve. Most of the time, people will, in general, lose confidence and resolve all through the diet. When that occurs, it is important to have someone to offer you the moral support you need to go on. If you have been eating vegetables the whole day and your family comes back home with a scrumptious chocolate cake and eats it before you, that will clearly not help at all.

As individuals, we need constant encouragement or else we are inclined to fail in achieving our objectives, paying little regard to their tendency. This is the reason your friends and relatives must be totally mindful of your plans and support your choice.

Lack of Ambition
Overweight people are in a continuous battle with the extra pounds because regardless of whether they figure out how to get rid of the extra weight and achieve a healthy weight, they need to fight to maintain the weight loss. This is where desire ventures in and plays an important role. Sadly, another reason why many people fail to stick to their diet is that they acknowledge defeat too easily and most times, surrender even before the battle begins. The reasons why this happens are many, but generally, they didn't have great motivation in the first place

Crash Dieting
The opposite of trend dieting - crash dieting - obviously mirrors our desire for instant gratification and the all too human reluctance to remain consistent.

However, it was the tortoise who beat the rabbit, and in dieting terms, the tortoise achieves the end goal, while the bunny wears himself out and resigns before the race is halfway through.

All too often, I meet high-strung people who positively believe that their bodies will instantly yoyo back to their earlier state after a period of dieting.

The major reasons why this occurs so frequently is because rather than following a long-term eating plan that can be customized for daily use (however, and I realize I constantly rumble like a broken record, it ought to be tied in with fixed new approaches and eating patterns), these characters go all out to lose all their excess weight in the shortest time possible, diving into semi-starvation trying to appease the desire for instant gratification.

Slow Metabolism
Many people face the problem of slow digestion, but this problem can be especially annoying for those who are on a weight loss diet. If you try a draconian diet and exhaust yourself at the gym, then at that point you definitely want to see some rewards for your effort. In any case, slow digestion translates to slow weight loss, and this is very demotivating for some. It is all about bodybuilding and the amount of time spent which can be a little while. Most surrender if they don't see the scale moving as much as they might want it to move.

Their Diets Do Not Provide Them With The Necessary Nutrients
Last, but not least, what most people fail to understand is that they should focus on a diet that gives them all the valuable nutrients that guarantee the best results. The diet must be

low in calories, not low in supplements and nutrients, minerals and amino acids which assume a significant role for your overall health and wellness. If you don't fuel your body appropriately, you will feel hungry all day and will eventually surrender and binge on food. Try not to think about your craving, as it tends to be most likely, your worst enemy.

Skipping Meals
Skipping meals isn't the fastest way to shed pounds. Some people think they can simply eat once every day and leave their body to burn off the fat. However, that is not how it works. When you skip a meal, your body goes into starvation mode. You're not getting the nutrients you need, and your body starts to slow down because it doesn't have the foggiest idea when it will get the necessary food once more. This frenzy causes your body to store all its fat, making it increasingly difficult to burn off. Your digestion starts to slow down to stop it from consuming and you stop losing weight. Which means, when you don't eat enough (under eat) you can put on weight because your body is turning into a vault and keeping the fat stored away safely within. Food is fuel. Eat when you're hungry. Quit eating when you are no longer hungry, not full.

Emotional Eating
Emotional Eating is a sensitive subject and a major problem with many people. Currently,

this doesn't imply that if you don't eat desserts when you're sad that you are not an over eater. If you snatch a sack of chips because you're exhausted or simply have a craving for something salty, or get frozen yogurt because you're focussed on, you are eating with your feelings. Comfort food is a term that accommodates emotional eating, which will in general climax around the holidays. In this way, making it increasingly difficult for those New Year's goals. About 75% of the people who binge do so is because they are emotional eaters. The main reason that you ought to eat is because you are hungry.

Unrealistic Expectation
A unique approach to dealing with most people, be it people fixing or some other, is to constantly undersell and over-deliver.

We all know that to do the reverse is to create distress and a nagging sense of disappointment. So why set yourself up for these negative, and damaging feelings by having desires that are generally unreasonable?

You may want a body like Brad Pitt or Oliver Proud lock, or even the muscular shapes and moves of a Lara Croft, but how about we get realistic for a moment. If you are 50lbs overweight and give yourself five weeks to get toned abs or tight buns, you are basically setting yourself up for disappointment. And with disappointment comes frustration, wrecking, and a slow (or swift) relapse back to your usual area of familiarity of unfortunate propensities and easy self-gratification.

Fad Dieting
In an age of marketing gimmicks and quick-fix solutions, the fad diet is the king of the dieting world.

The Grapefruit Diet, the Cabbage Diet, even the Atkins diet are, to be blunt, a waste of your time.

Anything that is short-term and unmaintainable, in other words, anything that doesn't instill new and long-lasting habits in your food intake, is in my view both a fad and counterproductive to your long-term achievement.

Chapter 3: How to change your displeasure into success in a healthy meal plan

Change in accordance with Your Taste Buds

If you don't like cauliflower, it won't work in your food plan. You can't force love (not in life and not in your food decisions). Obviously, you can attempt, but it either won't last or it won't be beneficial for you at last. One reason "diets" don't work is because we end up with plans set with foods that don't offer you an alternative. Great, whole foods are out there in numerous varieties so you don't need to plug your nose and swallow food you don't like. Discover one you do like and fill your food plan with those foods. Despise fish? Get your omegas from flaxseed oil. Try not to do servings of salads? Flare broil veggies. A war on food may get you to your objective for the time being, but it won't keep you there.

Factor in Your Activity Levels

Your daily exercises will also achieve your nutritional goals. The more active you are; the more calories you'll need to stay active. The less active you are, the less calories you need in the plan. Furthermore, activity levels help determine macronutrient requirements. As noted above, carbs, fats, and proteins are essential to help with building muscle, maintaining activity, or encouraging recovery. When you are making your ideal food plan, it is important that you consider these variables. When it comes to choosing your exercises and achieving your own health and wellness objectives, what you eat matters as much as the amount you eat.

Eat the Real Thing
Like relationships, when it comes to food, you want the real thing. You won't accept a friend who is not there for you or who supports you. So why would you say you are picking foods with artificial ingredients you can't pronounce? Real, whole foods have simple ingredients, have not been contacted by anything trying to make them different or been infused with anything to make them last more. They also use more energy to digest based on your body (Barr 2010). Real foods help you stay mentally alert; they stimulate you and support healthy digestion. There are a few warnings to stay away from "processed foods." Frozen strawberries, by definition, would be acceptable; However, I question why you would put Velveeta cheddar and a frozen strawberry in a similar classification. Staying away from highly processed foods is the way to a healthy food plan. Frozen veggies and fruits,

without any additives, are generally fine. Strawberry jam and butter wafers? All things considered, they should not appear in your shopping basket and pantry.

Keep it basic
Rather than being fixated on counting calories or measuring your portion sizes, think about your diet in terms of freshness, color, and variety. In addition, it ends up being easier to settle on healthy decisions. Begin by focusing on foods that you love and including some healthy fresh ingredients with them. Your diet will turn out to be significantly healthy and delicious in no time.

The key for a healthy diet is control
You may ask, what exactly is control and what's viewed as a moderate amount? That really depends on you, your body type, and overall dietary patterns.

Try focussing on balance. That typically will mean eating short of what you do now. For instance, if you have a burger for lunch, then you can have a healthy meal, for example, salmon and a serving of salad. If you eat 100 calories of chocolate one afternoon, you can adjust it by deducting 100 calories from your meal that night.

You'll want to incorporate a variety of starches, fat, fibre, protein, nutrients, and minerals to ensure that you maintain a healthy body.

Balance can also mean smaller portions. Serving sizes nowadays at eateries are incredibly enormous. When dining out, try part of an entrée with a friend. At home, use smaller plates. If you're still hungry after a meal, try including leafy green veggies or fruits.

Chapter 4: How to avoid making the same mistakes in a healthy diet plan

It is incredible that many people are starting to eat healthier – which is better for society, the earth, and everybody. However, as with anything new, it is easy to fail when you are just beginning. Here are 5 common slip-ups and confused arguments about healthy eating that you can easily stay away from:

Changing Your Diet Suddenly
Enthusiasm is good and it's never too soon to begin eating healthy but you need to do it gradually. An abrupt and drastic change in diet can present difficult challenges for your body. You may start to detox so rapidly that your body will most likely not know how to get rid of those poisons… the final product is that you harm yourself all at once. Also a list of potential side effects include– weakness, headaches, acid reflux, withdrawal symptoms, confusion, nausea.

Start slowly including healthy foods into your diet and gradually eat more of them and less of the usual foods you are used to. Before long, your diet will be changed and you will feel better as your body has time to process and adjust.

Overcooking Healthy Ingredients

You got yourself some natural vegetables and now you want to make a meal? That is an incredible beginning but the health benefit of vegetables and other foods is influenced by how you prepare them and how you eat them. For instance, boiling leafy greens significantly lessens the amount of vitamin C contained in them and heating nuts makes them harder to digest. Boiling vegetables that you will eat as sides also depletes a ton of the supplements which go into the water! Possibly boil vegetables when you will eat them together with the water they have been boiling in (for example – soups) else it is smarter to steam them.

Train yourself on the most effective way to handle healthy ingredients for the best results.

Cooking with Refined Olive Oil

Truly, olive oil is healthy because it is high in unsaturated fats and cell reinforcements. However, there is an obvious difference between normal, refined olive oil, and extra virgin olive oil. The latter has higher health and cell reinforcement values, minus the tons of artificial ingredients used in refinement. Moreover, extra virgin olive oil has high protection from oxidative weakening (loss of dietary benefit) because of the closeness of phenolic cancer prevention agents. These phenolic cell reinforcements are absent in refined olive oil, meaning that when you cook (bake/sauté/sear) with refined olive oil, the oil loses the advantages you thought you were getting.

Buy extra virgin olive oil. It is increasingly costly but you get a lot more in return! However, even extra virgin olive oil is altered when it achieves its smoking point – around 190°C, 375°F. Therefore, ensure that you cook your food at lower temperatures and use different oils for sautéing or high-heat cooking.

Opting for Skim Milk
Most people believe that all animal fat is bad. Therefore, it is easy to imagine that low-fat or zero-fat dairy is superior to whole milk and other dairy products. However, there are 2 fundamental factors that make low-fat milk a problematic choice:

1) Skim milk is often stacked with sugar – some normal 2-percent milk contains 12.3 grams of sugar! This is nearly as much as a chocolate chip cookie and Harvard researchers are forewarning that this substitution of sugar for fat may actually be a fundamental driver of weight-gain in many youngsters and grown-ups.

2) The nutrients contained in milk and dairy products are fat-soluble and, therefore, won't be consumed by your body except if you at the same time take inadequate amounts of fat.

If you love milk, try natural whole milk or nut milk. To get enough calcium, eat a greater amount of other extraordinary sources of calcium, for example, greens, nuts, and fish.

Over-depending On Supplements
There is not a viable alternative for healthy eating. Enhancements are only for that – enhancing a healthy diet, and ought to never turn into your essential source of nurtrients! Sadly, it is easy to see supplements as an alternate way to health – why experience the inconvenience of purchasing, cleaning, and eating fresh foods when you can take that powder container with your espresso?

The best (and most practical) approach to eating healthy is to eat more home-cooked meals prepared using fresh, natural ingredients. Cooking at home requires some serious energy but it doesn't need a great deal of investment! There are healthy meal plan administrations that deal with planning what to cook (including making plans for variety and richness of your diet), what to purchase and how to make a nutritious and tasty meal in less than 30 minutes. You can begin today by downloading a free 1-week meal plan.

Avoiding Healthy Fat
Have you at one point eaten a low-fat diet like spaghetti marinara just to wind up hungry within two or three hours? Eating a meal that doesn't have some fat, for example, cheddar or meat or healthy oils will unavoidably leave you feeling excessively hungry later. And that is a recipe for late-night bingers. Keep in mind, fat isn't the enemy. But choose your fats well and incorporate them as a major part of a controlled, nutritious diet.

So which are the key fats to choose? Monounsaturated fats (found in canola, nut, and olive oil) and polyunsaturated fats (found in sunflower, corn, and soybean oil) have been known to decrease "bad" cholesterol levels and increase "good" cholesterol.

Adding Extra Fat and Calories to Healthy Foods

What's the purpose of planning healthy dishes, like steamed veggies, just to stack them up with additional fat and calories from butter or cheddar? Without a doubt, even though you get similar supplements from the veggies, you're not helping your weight loss efforts. Your healthy serving of salads turns into a bad diet dream when you spread it with rich dressing.

Quit using normal salad dressing, cheddar, margarine, and mayo and you'll save more calories. You may even find that you prefer fresh or steamed veggies without the extras.

If you ideally can't stand the taste of plain vegetables, use herbs, flavors, Mrs. Dash, shower on butter, low-cal splash serving of salad dressings, salsa, or pico de gallo to add flavor to foods that you find bland.

Expecting Exercise Alone To Do The Trick
To shed pounds, you need to burn more calories than you consume. Basic math. Eventually, it doesn't make a difference if you're working out once—or even twice— each day, if you're eating too many fatty foods, you might surpass your daily allowance. You can become accountable by keeping a food and activity journal to know the number of calories you're consuming and burning.

Failure to Switch Up Your Workout Routine
In addition to the fact that it is exhausting, it's not particularly viable. If the main exercise you know is 30 minutes on the regular, you may not get the outcome you want. Surprise your muscles by changing the interval and force of your activity. Go for cardio a few times each week and weight-training exercises two times each week for maximum health and weight loss benefits. Crunched for time? You can spread the suggested 150 minutes of physical activity seven days into small lumps throughout the day. Studies show that short, 10-minute blasts of activity throughout the day can support your wellness and health. Consuming adequate protein, either by means of food or a protein

supplement, after working out can help amplify your muscle building results.

Neglecting A Diet Up Turn Into A Diet Spiral

We all surrender to the occasional unhealthy craving. To quickly address any feelings of blame, try not to castigate yourself when you fall off the wagon—simply recognize your oversight and refocus. Attempt to make it a learning experience. Consider what drove you astray and give careful consideration of it. Encourage yourself that one slip-up doesn't spoil all the work you've done.

Holding Back On The Good Stuff

You may believe you're getting all your required fruits and vegetables daily, but would you say you are really? You need about 2.5 quantities of vegetables and two quantities of fruits. Purpose to incorporate both in all your meals. Variety in your diet helps you get all the nutrients and supplements you need. Try different approaches to utilize fruits and vegetables into the food you eat—like making noodles from spiralizer zucchini or pizza outside layer from mixed cauliflower. You also might want to enhance with a multivitamin for added supplement support.

Chapter 5: Setting your personal goals

Set your objectives

When you are clear about your reasons for starting a healthy eating plan, it's a great time to set your objectives.

What is your long-term objective? A long-term objective is something you want to achieve in 6 months to a year. For instance, your long-term objective might be to:

- ➤ Lower your pulse and/or cholesterol.
- ➤ Reach a healthy weight for your body type.

What are the transient objectives that will enable you to achieve this? Short-term objectives are things that you want to do tomorrow and the following day. For instance, you may choose to:

- ➤ Switch to low-fat or skim milk or soy drink rather than whole milk with your cereal to reduce the amount of fat you take in.

- Cut back on eating fast food to once per week, or eat red meat just 3 times each week.
- Change a Habit by Setting Goals

Here are some clever tips about healthy eating objectives:

- Instead of changing your diet overnight, work on your improvements one at a time.
- Try adding something to your diet as opposed to removing something. Include foods that you think you need in greater quantities, like fruits and vegetables. If you begin off by removing things from your diet—like foods that are high in fat or sugar—you may feel deprived. And that will make it harder for you to change.
- Choose more healthy foods that you love. Make a list of the foods you like, and see how you can enhance them to make them healthier. For instance, make pizza at home using low-fat mozzarella cheddar and a batch of fresh vegetables. Is there a raw simple vegetable that you like? Stock up on it—and reach for it whenever you want a snack.

- Write down your objectives, and balance them up where you can see them. Going through your objectives can be a useful update.
- Don't set objectives that include shedding pounds fast. Quick weight loss isn't healthy and is difficult to maintain.

Track Your Progress

- Monitoring your progress makes you to realize how far you've come. It also makes you to continue with your plan.
- Use a note pad, diary, or food journal (What is a PDF report?) to monitor the healthy things you do. Go over it when you start to question yourself or feel deprived.
- Pay special consideration to how you feel. Are you able to see any difference when you are eating better? Or on the other hand, do you see any difference when you sometimes eat badly?
- Notice whether your food inclinations change. As we change what we eat, we figure out how to like new foods. You may find that you don't like a portion of the foods you used to eat before you began making changes in your diet. And you may have figured out how to like

new foods that you thought you didn't like.
- Look over any lab tests you may have if you are following a healthy diet. You may see improvements.
- Blood sugar tests will disclose to you whether your diet is controlling your diabetes.
- Periodic blood tests can reveal your cholesterol and triglyceride levels.
- You can check your circulatory strain to see whether dietary changes are improving it.
- High Blood Pressure: Checking Your Blood Pressure at Home
- Every time you reach an objective, reward yourself.

Consider your barriers

Make an effort to consider the things that could impede your success. We call these things barriers. And by considering them now, you can prepare for how to manage them if they occur.

Here are a few hints for managing barriers:

- It's absolutely normal to try something, stop it, and then get mad at yourself.

Most people need to attempt and attempt again before they achieve their objectives.

- If you have a desire for surrender, don't waste energy feeling bad about yourself. Keep in mind your reason for wanting to change, consider the achievements you've made, and give yourself a punch talk and congratulate yourself. Then, you may have a craving for healthy eating once more.
- When you hit a barrier—and many people do—get support. Talk with your relatives and friends to find out whether any of them wants to eat healthy with you or root for you.
- Don't overlook little rewards. Something to anticipate can keep you moving along.

Expect to experience a few obstacles. And remember: The thought isn't to get rid of obstacles but to identify them early and know what you will do to manage them.

It may help having a detailed personal activity plan (What is a PDF record?) where you list your objectives, your obstacles, and your plans to move beyond those barriers.

Get support—from others and from yourself

The more help you have, the easier it will be to change your dietary patterns.

Changing your lifestyle can appear to be overwhelming. However, when you know how to make just a couple of changes at once, it tends to be especially difficult to decide how to begin, or which change to make first. Your trainer can give you a referral to see a registered dietitian for nutrition training. This might be one plan or a continuation of plans to enable you to make sense of where you are currently and where you want to be. If you need some assistance, a dietitian can help you to set achievable objectives and offer direction and support as you change your lifestyle one small objective at a time.

If your relatives tell you that they love how you're getting healthier, you'll likely be propelled to keep doing better.

And there's more help out there. You can even ask for support.

Here are a couple of things to search for:

- Change your dietary patterns with a friend. It's encouraging to know that somebody has similar objectives. They can remind you how far you've come, and even propel you with what they have achieved.
- Friends and family might be an exceptional asset. Relatives can eat healthy meals with you and can encourage you by saying how they respect you for making hard changes. Friends may tell you how great you look because your dietary patterns have changed. Try not to be hesitant to tell family and friends that their support has a major effect on you.
- You may join a class or care group. People in these groups often have some of the same obstacles you have. They can give you support when you don't have a desire to continue with your eating plan and can support your resolve when you need a lift.
- Don't fail to reward yourself. When you achieve one of your objectives—for instance, eating five servings of leafy greens daily for several weeks—buy yourself a present. Purchase another healthy cookbook, take a cooking class,

or on the other hand, simply set aside some time for yourself. Take the necessary steps to encourage yourself that you've been meeting your objectives. You're fruitful!

Backing is everywhere. You simply need to search for it.

Check Your Weight

In the first place, find out where you are, which will help make sense of your nutritional objectives.

Weight is pervasive in America, and it is a risk factor for heart disease. One of the primary things to ask yourself before considering your diet is "Do I need to get in shape?" If you are overweight, losing 5 to 10 percent of your current weight can help bring down your risk for heart disease and diabetes. Determine your weight-related health risk by utilizing a Body Mass Indicator (BMI) Calculator.

Think about Calories

If you like to know your numbers, consider using a Calorie Calculator tool to gauge your calorie needs (Basic Metabolic Rate). Then, you will have a daily objective as a top priority, which can help when going through food names and keeping a definite food record.

Get Smart Goals

Defining small objectives that are attainable will help with achievement. And achievement breeds success. Before you know it, you'll be carrying on with a heart-healthier lifestyle and feel better about your accomplishments.

The best approach to ensure you are starting an eating plan that will be successful is to ensure your objectives are SMART, which is an abbreviation that stands for:

Specific	What do you intend to do? You may plan to walk more. But be more specific so the plan is clear. For instance, you intend to walk 20 minutes at lunchtime Monday through Thursday.
Measurable	You need to have the capacity to quantify your objectives to see your improvement. For instance, you might want to eat a serving of fruits or vegetables at every meal for several weeks.

	If you can mark it on your date-book or a journal, you can calculate it toward the week's end to know if you were able to increase your fruits or vegetables consumption.
Attainable	Don't make your objectives too difficult to reach. Make your objectives a progression of small advances so the ultimate objective is easier to accomplish. For instance, you might want to shed 20 pounds, but that takes a lot of hard work and time. You may get discouraged if you need to hold up that long to see any positive outcomes. Rather, you may set a feasible objective of losing 1 or 2 pounds each week by increasing your activity to 30 minutes 4 times each week and eliminating soft drinks. Finally, expand on this present objective's success with different objectives to achieve the 20-pound weight loss.

Realistic	Only define objectives you realize you will most certainly accomplish. That makes them practical. You may like dessert and feel you should set an objective that you'll never eat dessert again. But that is not a sensible objective. Rather try eating a ½ serving of frozen yogurt just on the weekends.
Time-oriented	Pick a timeline for achieving your objective. It has an end in sight, and ideally a short one. For instance, you realize that you need to keep a food journal to make sense of what you are eating. Set an objective to record all that you eat and drink for about fourteen days. Knowing it's not forever may help inspire you to achieve it.

Reward Yourself

It is an excellent idea to reward yourself for accomplishing your objectives. It will give you something to look forward to. It is ideal if the reward is something you possibly get if you complete your objective.

But don't use food as your reward. Try rewarding yourself with additional time spent with a friend, a diversion you've wanted to seek after or an activity that keeps you moving. Or on the other hand, attempt all three together! For instance, go walking with a friend and carry your camera to take photographs of nature, or take a running or yoga class out of the blue.

Chapter 6: The Meal Prep Fundamentals

Meal prep is the most vital thing an individual can achieve when trying to eat healthier foods. Indeed, when somebody asks me for weight loss guidance planning meals, it is the first thing we talk about.

Meal prep doesn't need to be something you fear. As opposed to making last minute basic supply trips and guessing the quantities, follow these 5 basic principles of effective meal prep!

For some individuals, meal prep has ended up being the way to achieving their wellness objectives. When they finally get the hang of it, their outcome hits the rooftop. Afterward, they'll often talk about it like it's the least difficult thing on the planet. "Better believe it, brother, take a couple of hours on Sunday and cook everything for the week."

Sadly, the entire process can prove overwhelming to the inexperienced, and even a significant hassle for the experienced. Hardly can seven days of meal prep take up a whole afternoon, but if fouled up, it can turn you off from the idea completely, and have you running for fast food on the regular.

Effective meal planning revolves around having a plan. This is vital. Try making things up along the way on the fly and you'll likely finish up with blundered macros, overcooked veggies, or, worse still, a foodborne illness. Before you even set foot in the kitchen, put these five meal prep principles to memory!

Pick Your Day Ahead of Time

Meal Prep Sunday is an occurrence widely seen in the wellness network. It might even be more famous than International Chest Day, otherwise known as Monday. Why? Preparing on the Sabbath doesn't interfere with your Friday and Saturday plans, and it's suitably close to the beginning of the week to (ideally) avoid having crazy smelling food by Thursday.

However, depending on the number of meals you're making, doing all the prep on a single day can mean a considerable amount of food and time. In addition, depending on your power of decision and favored cooking method, you may end up as that person or lady in the workplace known for their stinky lunches.

News flash: Meal prep is possibly going to last if it feels reasonable to you. If Sunday doesn't work, split meal prep into two days. This will eliminate the process length and undoubtedly protect the nature of your food. Sunday and Wednesday are usually a good pair, but identify any two days that work best for you.

Know Your Numbers

Try not to consider meal preparing until you know the exact amount you're shooting for as far as the number of meals involved and what those meals are made of.

Meals: Determine the number of meals and number of days you will plan at one time. Some people find that getting just their lunch ready for every day of the week is suitable, because they're ready to have breakfast and dinner at home. Others have more achievement preparing several every-day meals for the whole week—or even all of their meals. Regardless of where you fall on the meal preparing range, pick a day that sets you up for progress and plan in that manner.

Macros: If you're cycling carbs and you need 350 grams of carbs one day, but just 200 grams the following, know this early. Outline your everyday macros or needs, with specific meal by-meal rules, and post it somewhere in your kitchen. Where other than the fridge?

All things considered, you don't need to count macros to make this work. You can also use the "fist" strategy "to maintain a Caloric Deficit Without Counting Macros." But in either case, having strong rules early will ease the shopping and prep to come. You can even take it to the next dimension and mark containers by day and meal.

Stick With Staple Foods

So, investing energy creating gourmet mixtures, for example, crème brulee French toast or bacon-enveloped scallops in large quantities may keep you in the kitchen for a long time. Furthermore, generally speaking, the fancier something is, the worse it tastes when it has been lounging around for a couple of days in food containers.

Avoid the corruption for a new meal. When you're preparing, center around picking easy-to-cook, pre-packaged foods that store well. My proposal is to mix and match from these classifications and get down to business:

- ➢ Protein: Chicken breast, lean ground hamburger, pork tenderloin, flank steak,

lean lunch meat (turkey breast, ham, or roast meat) and low-fat hamburger jerky
- ➢ Carbohydrates: Oats, quinoa, couscous, darker rice, wild rice, entire grain tortillas, and bread
- ➢ Healthy fats: Almonds, walnuts, pecans, pistachios, pumpkin seeds, nutty spread, almond butter, olive oil, and coconut oil

I'm not a fish fellow when it comes to ready meals, but don't hesitate to explore. Simply ensure you use an all-around fixed holder!

Go Grocery Shopping

Shopping for food may appear painfully obvious, but starting your meal prep with leftovers is never a smart idea. Indeed, you may get a meal or two that way, but eventually, you'll either come up short on food or will be forced to use your protein-powder stash as fortifications—for almost each meal. That gets costly fast.

When you know your numbers, ensure you have everything to meet them. If you're one of those lucky people with a chest fridge, you will almost certainly prepare on time. If not, make a weekly or every other week trip a part of your prep schedule. Not only will it help you skillfully explore the store, but it will also enable you save extra money and avoid food waste.

Put Money into A Fridge or Insulated Meal Bag

The idea of the refrigerator having your meals for the week is quite pleasing. In fact, Instagram concurs. Towers of Tupperware neatly stocked with the ideal mix of macros—man, it's a sight to see! But come Monday morning, you'll have a difficult time carrying your duffel bag, briefcase, and various containers to work. A lot of undeserving meals have wound up on the ground this way.

If you're preparing only one meal per day, you'll most certainly swing it. If you're the, a few meals a day sort, then a fridge, protected meal pack, or rucksack of some sort is necessary. Their controlled temperature can also help shield you from foodborne diseases.

This additional purchase may seem like an extravagance, but it has the potential to spare you a lot of daily disappointments. If you do this well—which is the best way to do it—then eliminating unnecessary hassles is necessary! Make it easy, make it yours, and make it last.

Chapter 7: Tips To Make Meal Prep Easier And Faster

Make a Plan
Make a list of your favorite healthy foods, to pick simple recipes that can be made quickly or in bulk, and choose what you'll eat for each snack and meal. This approach will get easier and faster with training. If you're following the 21 Day Fix or want to use its simple methodology, you can download its meal plan tools here.

Star Tip: Save your preparation for a future week. When you have a couple of meal prep menus in your possession, you can turn to them to keep things interesting.

Mix Things Up
It very well may tempt simply eating similar meals consistently, but you'll eventually get exhausted. Meal prep master Amanda Meixner suggests no less than two lunch alternatives and two meal choices. This can be as simple as picking different proteins for your salads every day or eating chicken with vegetables three evenings of the week, and fish or tofu with vegetables the other two. When you get the

hang of it, you can get increasingly creative with your recipes.

Search for Shortcuts
Purchase pre-cut veggies and fruits, cooked lentils, or rotisserie chicken. Fish is an easy no-cook protein to add to servings of salads or snacks. As of now, have your oven on to roast veggies? Why not attempt this tip for cooking twelve eggs without a moment's delay from @choose_you_fitness? Preheat your oven to 325°, then put your eggs in a biscuit tin and bake them for 30 minutes. Then, cautiously remove them and dump the eggs into a bowl of ice water until cool. Are you inclined toward the normal approach? Here's our way to deal with perfect hard-boiled eggs.

Jump on the Mason Jar Salad Bandwagon
Mason container plates of salads are the sweethearts of Pinterest and Instagram because they're pretty, but they're also useful. They cost about a dollar a piece, are microwave safe (simply make sure to remove the top), and can be used for different kinds of meals. Their vertical shape makes them especially pleasant for storing salads. Since the dressing is at the base of the container, and the salads at the top, nothing gets spongy!

Put money into Food Storage Containers
A small investment in food containers of different sizes to suit your needs will improve things greatly. It's a smart idea to pick one container type and purchase a few that pile and store conveniently. If you pick plastic containers, ensure they are without BPA and that they won't melt in the microwave or dishwasher. Strong Pyrex dishes with covers are also extraordinary as are Mason containers. If you choose to bet everything on the meal prep lifestyle, you may want to consider getting a protected pack to carry your meals everywhere you go.

Keep Snacks Simple
When you're cooking everything for the week on the double, it's critical to keep things simple. Spare time by picking snacks that don't require a ton of time to put together. Fresh fruits, hard-boiled eggs, and pre-cut veggies with prepared hummus are incredible choices.

Cook Foods All at Once
Roasting vegetables, sweet potatoes, and even chicken breasts all at once will spare you time, and cut down on your service bill. Envision... all of your side dishes for the week... prepared in around 30 minutes!

Stick to Your Grocery List
Try not to let poor-quality food sneak into your shopping basket. Not having it in the house implies not making use of your self-discipline to keep away from it. Want to make a drive purchase? If you can figure out how to fit it into your eating plan for the week, pull out all the stops. Simply keep these to a minimum so that nothing goes to waste. By sticking to your list and by limiting the spur of the moment purchases, you'll save extra money.

Remember About Shakeology
Especially if you have an inclination that you're short on fruits, this is one healthy snack to go with!

Keep Your Eyes on the Prize
All of this meal prep is for a reason... to enable you to achieve your health and wellness objectives. When clean eating is as basic as reaching into the fridge for your lunch or dinner, you'll be less tempted to stop for fast food or request takeout. Regardless of whether you do your meal prep for the week, all at once, or only a couple of days on end, doing so will enable you to stick to your meal plan and give you more opportunity to Push Play!

Chapter 8: Kitchen Tools We Need For Meal Prep

Preparing and cooking portions (or all) of your meals a few days before you intend to eat them is an essential technique to save time and energy during busy weekdays. It's also a clever way to save extra money. (We are certain, in any case, that the fine people at your neighborhood sushi eatery will be sad to not see you so frequently.)

While #MealPrepSunday might be en vogue at this moment, it has for some time been the passionate cook's—and eatery chef's—mystery weapon. After all, if you can knock out all of the cleaving, mixing, and pre-cooking on the double, and spare yourself the hassle later, you most certainly should.

Instant Pot
I realize this device is all the rage in the health world of late, but it's in light of current circumstances. I got one a few years back for Christmas and have just as of late begun using it to meal prep – and let me tell you, it's been a definite benefit. It's great for quickly cooking things like soup or bone stock and it's also amazing for clump cooking things like rice,

beans, shredded chicken . . . and so on. My favorite Instant Pot recipe right now? This Butternut Lentil Turkey Chili is SO yummy!

Slow Cooker
Before I bought a pressure cooker, my programmable slow cooker was my mystery weapon for meal prep, and despite everything, it makes the cut! It's so easy to toss ingredients in the slow cooker at the start of the day and have a delectable, healthy meal prepared to eat by day's end. I also value it for making slow cooker cereal. Psst . . . stay tuned for some slow cooker meal prep fridge meals – healthy eating has never been so easy!

Spiralizer
Spiralizers make vegetables extra tasty and feel increasingly generous in a meal. Substitute your pasta for certain zucchini "noodles", or use spiralizer apples for a healthy alternative of crusty fruit-filled treat. I know stores are selling prepared veggie noodles nowadays, but it's less expensive to make your own. I value my spiralizer for making zoodles, sweet potato noodles, broccoli noodles and more. Try spiraling with these recipes: Zucchini Noodle Lo Mein and Zucchini Noodle Ramen.

Serving of Salad Chopper Bowl
You know my love for the salad chopper bowl. It is the way to uniformly cut and mix servings of salads. You can prepare your salad ingredients early (keep the dressing as an afterthought) and then when it's time to eat, just prepare all of your salad ingredients and dressing in the salad chopper bowl and cut away! The outcome is a splendidly chopped eatery quality plate of salad.

Mason Jars
Incredible for overnight oats, chopped veggies with reducing sauce on the bottom, or Mason container salad, this powerhouse stockpiling holder will make your meal prep fun.

Food Processor
Food processors have such a significant number of uses – I use it for crushed veggies, cauliflower rice, sauces, salsa, and energy balls/bars. Give it a shot with these poultry food energy chomps.

Mason or Weck Jars
If you're new to meal prep, Mason or Weck containers are perfect-size containers, to begin with. They're modest and can store almost anything! I love the wide mouth Ball Mason containers for salad and use smaller 16 ounces or ½ half quart containers for overnight oats.

A Good Set of Knives
Try not to hate on my affection for good, sharp knives. If you haven't bought yourself a good set of knives, trust me, it's necessary, despite all the trouble! Cleaving is a lot easier and more practical when you have great knives. I adore our Shun knives, but I was also gifted a few knives from Material that are superb, and come in charming hues and are quite inexpensive.

Extraordinary Set of Knives
Cleaving, chopping, and mincing vegetables and herbs is a lot easier (and more secure!) with sharp cutting knives. Put money into a good set, and you won't regret it—we guarantee! (Got a set you love that are getting dull? Find out how to keep them sharp!)

Biscuit Tin and Silicone Muffin Liners
I enjoy making egg biscuits, oat biscuits, and protein biscuits to reach for easy breakfasts and snacks constantly. Silicone biscuit containers are extremely easy to clean . . . and if you know how irritating biscuit tins can be to clean, you know these are unquestionably #worthit.

Measuring Cups and Spoons
Another fundamental when it comes to meal prep! I love these bright containers and

spoons, and they have attractive handles so they remain intact and are easy to wash (simply toss them in the dishwasher).

Zip Top Baggies
While glass stockpiling containers are perfect for storing prepared meals, they're not generally the most reliable. You'll want to keep a couple of different sizes of fridge safe zip-top bags around for storing snacks to go, or freezing smaller amounts of prepared foods.

Fluid Measuring Cups
It's incredible to have a fluid measuring container on hand. I use it for . . . you got it, measuring any fluids! It's more accurate and it's easier to pour the fluid using these measuring containers.

Food Scale
If you're prone to waste, this is a wonderful device to take your meal prep to the next level. A few recipes have weight requirements so it's nice to have around – especially if you're a baker. Food scales also prove to be useful if you're learning portion sizes or following your food selection.

Spicer
This kitchen tool may appear to be a one-trap horse, but it's more versatile than you think. In

addition to spicing citrus for marinade, salad dressings, and sauces, you can make speedy work of "mincing" garlic and ginger, as well as finely grinding cheddar or even hot peppers.

Kitchen Scale
So as to guarantee you're receiving the right nutrients, you'll want to know exactly how much food you're eating. While measuring mugs will work fine for vegetables, beans, and grains, a kitchen scale is useful for measuring out your proteins. Look for a computerized scale that can measure in grams and ounces for more accuracy.

Preparing or Roasting Sheet Pans
I love my cooking stove but you can run with any type of baking sheets. I like using non-rimmed sheet searches for gold like cookies, but the rimmed ones are best for roasting veggies and sheet dish meals. If there happens to be any fluid discharged during cooking, the edge guarantees it doesn't dribble all over your oven and make major chaos.

Glass Storage Containers
Try not to waste time with plastic storing containers. Put money into glass ones. They're sheltered from synthetic compounds, won't twist in the dishwasher, and go from the fridge

to the microwave—no need to grimy up another plate.

Search for a collection of food containers; they'll likely be a superior type than individual containers. Get a couple of glass containers, too. Small ones (4-oz containers) are incredible for salad dressing and sauces. Bigger ones are perfect for to-be-mixed smoothie ingredients, overnight oats, and soups.

Casserole Dishes
9×13 is the standard size for casseroles, so I would get that kind – but it's also good to have a square casserole dish (either 8×8 or 9×9). This Pyrex set has the two sizes and comes with a cover for each.

Portion Pan
Ideal for making quick breads like banana bread or exquisite dishes that come in portion structure like my vegetarian lentil portion.

A Great Set of Pots and Pans
I'm a major enthusiast of artistic non-stick skillets. I have an assortment of sizes for different uses and I use them every day! One thing to note is that they do in general, lose their non-stick attributes before long – usually not more than a year. All things considered, they're not overly costly and they're something

I use each day, so I'm alright with buying new ones consistently. For pots, I have these two Calphalon non-stick pots and adore them. I also have a vast Le Creuset cast-iron round dutch oven that I use for soups and stews.

Stackable Lunch/Bento Box
Pre-pack lunches during meal prep and you can get and go during the week. Bento boxes allow you to partition things in discrete containers to keep things new.

Silicone Baking Cups
Essential for anticipating make-ahead breakfast recipes like biscuits and egg mugs, these silicone glasses are also incredible for storing food and snacks in lunch boxes.

Cutting Boards
Pretty much every recipe you turn to will include some cleaving, cutting, dicing, and so on, so this tool ought to be close at all times! You can pick plastic or wood. In any case, we suggest having one board for your vegetables and another for slicing meat to avoid cross-contamination

Mixing Bowls

Mixing bowls aren't only used for heating recipes like baked cereal, they can be used for everything from making meatballs, marinating proteins, making dressings and also storing salads for a quick snack and go to lunch! We like to use treated steel or a strong plastic set that comes in 3-5 pieces. We picked the glass bowls because they are easy to clean, dishwasher safe, and look great on camera when you're making those tasty style food recordings.

Colander
From reducing pasta to draining beans, fruits, and vegetables, this kitchen tool will make it easy to eat new, fresh produce! Say goodbye to poor artificial mixtures and hello to fresh rainbow veggies! You can settle on a tempered steel or plastic one.

Silicone Baking Mats
Silicone heating mats are an ideal, reusable approach to line your sheet skillet to shield food from staying. They're non-harmful and dishwasher safe, too. Preparing a huge bunch of roasted veggies is a lot easier when nothing sticks to the skillet!

Fine Mesh Stainless Steel Strainers
A lot of strainers make washing a breeze. Use them to wash berries, grapes, veggies, and the like so they're prepared to go for the week.

They're also essential for washing whole grains like brown rice and quinoa before cooking. Put the flushed grains to use by cooking a large batch and then using in dishes and salad.

Stainless Steel Canning Funnel
This little channel makes filling Mason containers with pre-packed ready meals too fast and easy. A small kitchen basic that makes prep so much easier!

Chapter 9: How to go BPA free

Bisphenol-A (BPA) has gotten a ton of negative press to such an extent, that another enactment was as of late introduced to boycott food packages containing BPA. But there's no need to hold up until the administration gets around to forbidding the stuff. Make do with a BPA –free kitchen using these simple tips.

If you should use plastic, search for those items marked BPA-free. Refrain from using plastic containers that contain the reuse codes 3 or 7, numbers which indicate that they might be made with BPA.

Toss old, scratched plastic water bottles. Use of plastic synthetic substances might be better when the surface is worn out.

Refrain from microwaving plastic containers or placing them in the dishwasher except if they are marked microwave-and dishwasher-safe.

Try not to reuse single-use plastics. When used over and again, they can separate and release synthetic compounds.

Settle on glass, porcelain, or treated steel containers, especially for hot food or fluids.

(KleanKanteen and Hydro Flask make tempered steel water bottles.)

Search for foods sold in BPA-free jars (Eden Foods is one brand that offers them) or BPA-free containers (Pomì, maker of tomato items, and Pacific are two organizations that use such parts).

➢ Drink faucet water or use BPA-free treated steel water bottles (from organizations like Nalgene or Sigg) rather than slugging down filtered water. Difficulty Rating: Easy
➢ Instead of eating microwavable meals that leave plastic boxes, eat just freshly prepared, natural foods. Difficulty Rating: Moderate (or hard, depending on where you live, the amount in your bank account, and how apathetic you are).
➢ Instead of using plastic utensils, rely on the more drawn out lasting collection. Difficulty Rating: Easy
➢ To stay protected, stay away from all canned foods and replace with non-canned varieties (supplant canned soup with soup in a container, for instance) except if jars mean that they have a BPA-free lining. If that is impractical, stay

away from these specific canned foods, which are known to be high in BPA: coconut milk, soup, meat, vegetables, meats, juice, fish, beans, meal substitution beverages, and fruits (indeed, we understand that includes most canned foods). Take special consideration to stay away from foods that are acidic, salty, or greasy. Difficulty Rating: Hard

➢ Steer clear of plastic storage containers for left-over food. Rather, use glass containers that come with BPA-free plastic covers. The food ought not to come into contact with the tops. Difficulty Rating: Easy

➢ Instead of using a plastic coffee maker or going out for espresso, use a French press or clay dribble. Difficulty Rating: Moderate (if you like to drink your espresso during the workday)

Regardless of whether you follow all of these means, BPA will unavoidably be found in your body; hints of it are found in extremely unlikely places, for example, whole eggs and milk (due to pre-showcase preparing). But a considerable number of these recommendations will prompt a healthier lifestyle. Regardless, there's little damage to eating fresh food, staying away from filtered water, and curbing the impulse for espresso purchases. There's no damage in trying, and surely no mischief in reducing the harmful poisons in your body. Except if you're into that kind of thing.

Know Your Plastics

You can easily assume that dark plastics are free of BPA. In this way, if you can't see through it, that is the initial step in identifying BPA-free plastics in your home.

For any plastics that fit the description of being hard, clear (or clear-tinted) and unbreakable, flip them over and search for a re-using number. Polycarbonate plastics will have a number 7 on them, but they're not by any means the only plastic that gets marked with a 7, so you'll need to do more exploring.

Hope to check whether the container is named as unbreakable or microwave-safe. If it is, that is a good pointer that it contains BPA. Get rid of it.

If you see a name suggesting that the holder is hand wash, it's likely made of acrylic and, therefore, OK to keep.

If the holder doesn't have a re-using number on it and you got it before July of 2012, it's ideal to assume that it contains BPA and to dispose it.

Metal containers, especially aluminum water bottles, are at times lined in BPA to improve the taste of the water. If you feel any plastic coating inside a container that isn't set apart as BPA-free, it's advisable to discard it. These sorts of linings are especially inclined to scratch.

Safety

Polycarbonates get a great deal of bad press because of worries over BPA, but remember that it isn't the main plastic that can filter synthetic compounds into your food. While you're feeling your plastic containers, feel free to throw any that are scratched or damaged. Worn compartments represent a higher draining danger.

Other filtering dangers include:

- Microwaving food in plastic containers
- Storing acidic foods (like tomato sauce) in plastic because the causticity could draw synthetic substances into your food

- Placing foods in containers while they're as yet hot
- Scrubbing containers too energetically or with scrubbers that can cause scratches
- Routinely exposing your containers to high temperatures, including washing them in the dishwasher
- Using containers over an extensive period.

A smart approach is to change to using glass in your kitchen; you won't need to stress over any of these worries because glass:

- Is microwave-safe
- Is dishwasher-safe
- Won't recolor
- Doesn't wear out
- Won't drain chemicals into your food if it progresses toward becoming scratched or is exposed to high temperatures

Chapter 10: How to Store Different Types of Foods

Putting away foods can present its own kind of issues. And different kinds of foods have different capacity prerequisites to keep bacteria from setting in. Here are some tips to protect your family and yourself.

Storing Vegetables

1. Vegetables ought to be stored in the vegetable crisper in the fridge. However, keep potatoes, sweet potatoes, onions, and garlic in a cool, dull, all around ventilated spot, but not in the fridge. Tomatoes have better flavor if they are not refrigerated. When cut, tomatoes ought to be refrigerated like any vegetable.

2. Store vegetables in the fridge crisper in plastic bags to avoid loss of dampness and dietary benefits. Eggplant and capsicums ought to be kept open in the crisper as they sweat if stored in plastic bags. Place mushrooms in a paper sack (not in a plastic pack) before setting them in the crisper.

Putting away Fruits

3. Apples and berries ought to be kept in the fridge for freshness. Summer fruits ought to sit at room temperature until they are ready, and then go into the fridge. Grapes and fruits that are not entirely ready can be left in a fruit bowl in the kitchen.

4. Citrus fruits are fine at room temperature except if it is hot, in which case, place them in the fridge.

Bananas ought to be kept at cool room temperature. Their skins become dark if they are refrigerated. However, they are still fine to eat.

Putting away Dairy Products

5. Regularly check the expiry date on dairy products, especially milk. Try not to purchase milk if it will expire in 2-3 days. Milk generally begins by giving off a smell before its expiry date regardless of whether you store it in the fridge! Generally, milk bottles at the front of the rack in the market have an expiry date of just a couple of days. Search for containers at the back of the rack.

Putting away Frozen Foods

6. Pack all your frozen foods together in a protected bag to keep them frozen until you return home. If foods defrost on the way home and you re-freeze them in a residential fridge, massive ice crystals will form and can crack cell layers in the food allowing nutrients to get away. Keep frozen foods for quality, as bacteria will start to multiply when the food is defrosted.

Putting away Meat Products

7. New meat, chicken, and fish have a few bacteria so these foods should be kept frozen. Bacterial growth slows down in the fridge; at room temperature, they develop quickly. Cooking executes these bacteria. Store meat, seafood, and chicken in the coldest section of the fridge. See that any uncooked items don't come into contact with different foods in the fridge. They ought to be put away at the bottom part of the fridge so that any juices that leak out won't contaminate different foods on lower racks.

8. Ensure that fish or other seafood are wrapped and used at once. Throw them out if not used within two days.

9. If you are going to freeze meat, seafood, or poultry, enclose it in fridge wrap and freeze without a moment's delay after bringing it home. Store eggs in the fridge, ideally in their containers, as it provides protection and prevents dampness loss through the shell.

Putting away Other Products

10. Try not to allow pet foods to come into contact with human foods. Storeroom things (canned foods, oats, and so on) ought to be put away in a dark place like in cupboard or pantry. Keep oils out of direct light.

Chapter 11: Food Hygiene Tips for Your Fridge

Keep in mind that your fridge ought to be set at a temperature between 0-5°c with the goal that the rate of food decay is slowed and harmful bacteria can't multiply. At this temperature, your food will remain safe to eat.

Also, ensure you watch out for use-by dates. Any food that has passed its use-by date ought not to be eaten as harmful bacteria has had the opportunity to develop and make the food risky to health. Foods past their best-before dates can be eaten as this is just a sign of value, not welfare.

General Rules of Refrigeration

> - Ensure that the fridge is never overburdened. While packing that last bit of food into the fridge may seem like a smart idea at the time, you are in threat of blocking the cooling unit that will cool your food. There is also a threat that the refrigerator won't close, making your food unfit to eat the next morning! Air needs to have the ability to flow around the food.

- New stock ought to be set behind old stock. Indeed, the rules in a business kitchen ought to apply at home as well. Ensure you eat the food in the fridge based on the use by date so as to avoid food wastage which eventually hits your wallet!
- Open jars ought to never be put away in the fridge as this may result in concoction pollution, especially acidic food, for example, fruits. If you wish to put canned food in the ice chest, guarantee that you put the food into a holder that is reasonable for chilling first.
- If your fridge temperatures are too high, it might be the result of over-burdening, the obstructing of cooling units, or the indoor regulator being set too high. If your fridge does not have a thermometer inside, we suggest that you purchase a fridge thermometer to screen the temperature. Remember that the right temperature is-0-5°c.

Take special consideration with high-risk foods

Food-harming bacteria can develop and increase in certain kinds of food more easily than others. High-risk foods include:

- Raw and cooked meat, including poultry, for example, chicken and turkey, and foods containing them, for example, casseroles, curries, and lasagne.
- Dairy products, for example, custard and dairy-based desserts like custard tarts and cheesecake.
- Eggs and egg products, for example, mousse.
- Small goods, for example, hams and salamis.
- Seafood, for example, seafood serving of mixed greens, patties, fish balls, stews containing seafood, and fish stock.
- Cooked rice and pasta
- Ready salads like coleslaws, pasta salad, and rice salad.
- Ready fruits salad.
- Ready-to-eat foods, including sandwiches, rolls, and pizzas that contain any of the food above.

Food that comes in bundles, jars, and containers can turn out to be high-risk foods once opened, and ought to be handled and stored correctly.

Storing cooked food safely

When you have cooked food and want to cool it:

- ➢ Put hot food into shallow dishes or smaller parts to help cool the food as fast as possible.
- ➢ Don't put extremely hot food into the fridge. Hold up until steam has stopped emanating from the food before placing it in the fridge.

Avoid refreezing defrosted food

Food-harming bacteria can develop in frozen food while it is defrosting, so refrain from defrosting frozen food in the temperature threat zone. Keep defrosted food in the refrigerator until it is ready to be cooked. If using a microwave to defrost food, cook it after defrosting.

When in doubt, avoid refreezing defrosted food. Food that is frozen a second time is likely to have larger amounts of food-harming bacteria. The risk relies upon the state of the food when frozen, and how the food is handled between defrosting and refreezing, but raw food ought to never be refrozen once defrosted.

Store raw food separately from cooked food

Raw food and cooked food ought to be put away separately in the fridge. Bacteria from raw food can contaminate cold cooked food, and the bacteria can increase to dangerous levels if the food isn't cooked all at once.

Continuously store raw food in firm or secured containers at the base of the refrigerator. Keep raw foods beneath cooked foods, to maintain a strategic distance from fluid, for example, meat squeezes dripping down and contaminating the cooked food.

Pick strong, non-toxic food storing containers

Ensure your food storing containers are perfect and in great condition, and just use them for putting away food. Cover them with tight-fitting covers, foil or plastic film to limit potential contamination. Exchange the element of opened jars into appropriate containers.

If in hesitation, throw it out

Throw out high-risk food left in the temperature threat zone for over four hours – don't place it in the fridge and don't keep it for an extended time. Check the use-by dates on food items and dispose of obsolete food. If you are skeptical of the use-by date, toss it out.

Chapter 12: Purchasing Exact Amounts of Food to Save Time and Money

Holding the expense down
Regardless of whether it's grabbing the basics like bread and milk, having some espresso around the local area or discovering lunchbox fillers for the children, looking for food is something many of us do almost daily and the expense can easily go up! We as a whole want to discover great quality, healthy food at moderate costs, so look at our tips to learn how you can get more for your money...

At home
Keep a store cabinet of durable things such as pasta, rice, soups, noodles, wafers, crispbreads, oatcakes, flour, corn flour, canned vegetables, such as tomatoes and sweetcorn, kidney beans, baked beans, canned sleek fish (for example sardines, fish, mackerel), tomato puree, soy sauce, Worcestershire sauce, pepper, herbs, flavors, garlic and ginger.

Before you shop - Plan.
- ➢ Set your financial plan for food
- ➢ Plan your meals for the week

- ➢ Make a shopping list

General Shopping Tips
- ➢ Don't shop on an empty stomach!
- ➢ Stick to your shopping list and stay away from spur of the moment purchases.
- ➢ Do a major weekly/monthly bulk shopping and an everyday trip for foods that have a short timeframe of realistic usability, such as milk.
- ➢ For bigger households, purchase in bulk, for example, large bags of potatoes.
- ➢ Check out grocery stores' own brands – they are less expensive and the quality is equally as great. Look at marks on items for salt, fat and sugar levels. Become familiar with food marks here.
- ➢ When contrasting brands, take a gander at the weight you get at the cost.
- ➢ Look for special offers – but be careful. It's a deal if it's something you needed in the first place and if you can use it. A few things can be frozen in smaller quantities so that you can defrost when needed.
- ➢ Supermarkets often sell food inexpensively toward the day's end – however, check the use by dates.

- If possible, look around. It might be more practical to go to a grocery store when completing an extensive shop.
- If purchasing desserts, chocolate or crisps, limit to maybe a couple of days out of each week. Purchasing multi-packs might be more practical and offer smaller part sizes.

Meat, Fish, and Eggs
- By purchasing meat in a butcher's shop or at the meat counter in a grocery store, you get the opportunity to pick the exact amount you want. As a guide, a serving of meat is normally about 2oz (60g) each – the span of a large portion of a chicken breast, or the palatable segment of a sheep hack.
- Mince-meat is of great value, versatile, and has minimal waste. But it very well may be high in fat. A good tip is to purchase a smaller amount of slimmer (and better quality) mince and build up your dish with vegetables.
- Fish cooks quickly and is really nutritious. Mackerel, coley, herrings, fish fingers and tinned fish are all great incentives for money.
- Eggs are a great value, easy to cook, and loaded with goodness. Boil, poach, or

scramble your eggs for the healthiest outcome.

Fruits, vegetables, and potatoes
- Fruit and vegetables can be less expensive in green merchants than in the general store.
- Potatoes are flexible – steam, boil, mash, roast, or make your very own potato wedges or chips. This is less expensive than purchasing ready mash, wedges, or chips.
- Buy foods in season.
- Include some frozen, dried or tinned alternatives- they all check towards your 5-a-day. Pick fruit canned in its very own juice, not syrup and of course search for the alternative with minimal sugar and salt when picking tinned foods.
- Frozen vegetables are super because there's no waste with them. And because they're frozen soon after they're picked, they're normally brimming with flavor too.
- Remember when you purchase pre-packaged fruits and vegetables, you are paying for the packaging.
-

When cooking
- Eating prepared meals and other foods can be costly and they can contain large amounts of concealed fat/salt/sugar. Home-cooked options are more nutritious and usually more affordable.
- Bulk up stews, casseroles, and different dishes using extra vegetables and pulses. This will allow you to reduce the amount of meat needed. These can be purchased dried or in jars. Make sure to carefully stick to the cooking and drenching directions.
- If utilizing tomato-based pasta sauce, use a tin of tomatoes as an economical method for making the sauce go further.
- Base your meals around boring foods, for example, potatoes, rice, and pasta. These foods are inferior and nutritious.
- Check your use by dates on the things in your fridge/cabinets. Many of us waste huge quantities of food because it expires before we can use it. Plan your meals so that everything gets eaten or frozen for some time later.
- Cook once – eat twice! Make extra when cooking foods, for example, curries, stews, and soups, and freeze the rest in separate containers. These can be useful

for lunches or on nights when you don't have a great deal of time.

At work
- Invest in a lunchbox and make your own sandwiches at home to carry to work – you'll spare a fortune!
- If you normally pay for tea or espresso during your working day, why not invest in a flask and bring along your very own portion? Custom made soup will also remain hot for the day in a flask.
- Fill a cleaned jug with crisp faucet water every day and carry this to work as opposed to purchasing filtered water.
- Bring a lunchbox to work. Fill an impenetrable lunchbox with healthy snacks, for example, fruits, nuts or home-made popcorn and keep around your work area for when hunger strikes.

Chapter 13: Vegan Cooking Tips and Tricks

There is a huge deal of confusion that vegan food is exhausting. In my mind, nothing could be further from the truth, but I do concur. There are my Top 10 vegan cooking tips and tricks. Here are a couple of my top choices:

Serve this Green Monster Hummus with saltines or pita bread at your next family meal. **Olive Oil** – Even adding only a little bit of olive oil can really draw out a dish. Clearly, it's easy to go overboard on this. I've discovered that a little spot will do, but I do love the flavors it includes. I've use olive oil on Hummus, Pastas, and even cakes!

Spice Girls – Don't fear your spice rack. A friend gave me an incredible tip once. She said to put the spice on your tongue so you know what you're adding to a dish before you do it. Don't simply rely on a recipe to tell you what to add to your food. I want to have smoked paprika, garlic powder, cinnamon, turmeric, dill, ginger, nutmeg, caraway seeds, and allspice close by more often than not. I also grow fresh herbs like basil, oregano, sage, and parsley. I include flavors like rosemary and sage to roasted potatoes. It has such an effect.

Citrus it up – It's a smart idea to keep a lemon or lime close by because citrus is an extraordinary taste enhancer. You'll also get a touch of nutrient C in your diet. In addition, having a little lemon on hand to add to your tea is unquestionably good! Or on the other hand, what about lime for your margarita? Now we're talking. Also, I learned from my friend Liz that crushing a little bit of lemon over your salad is an extraordinary, fresh (and super-low calorie) dressing. Who knew?

Nuts and Seeds – OK. So there is some fact to the entire crunchy granola side of veganism. But the thing is, nuts and seeds are SO bravo! I love adding nuts to my smoothies to include a rich surface. I also add them to veggie burgers for the additional fat they give. I'm a major devotee of hemp seeds as well. And, obviously, we use flax seeds in a lot of our recipes.

Three cuts of dark bean brownies are stacked over one another with a bowl of chocolate chips behind them. Beans, Beans, Good for the heart! We generally have beans on hand, regularly. We keep them dried and canned. We use canned beans more often than not, but I also like having the dried variety around. Our most loved beans are dark beans but we also use chickpeas, pinto beans, and kidney beans. And in some cases, it's only enjoyable to attempt different sorts of beans to mix things up. You can't deny the astounding flavor and healthy fibre in each nibble! I've even used beans in my Black Bean Brownies.

Make it Savory – Here are five of my favorite things to add to a recipe to make an exceptional portion appetizing: a) We, generally keep vegetable stock close and use it as a seasoning in soups and stews. b) White wine. I may state red wine here, but I think white wine is more versatile. I add it to soups or even things like stew when I want a special portion of exquisite. c) Tomatoes. Take a stab at making minestrone without tomatoes. It simply doesn't work. It might sound insane, but however, adding a jar of stewed tomatoes to a vegetable soup gives it a kind of buttery flavor. We keep stewed, diced, and sun-dried tomatoes around all the time. And we even try to have tomato sauces and pastes as well. d) Adding a little bit of Mild Miso Paste to your recipe can have a major effect and finally, e) I suggest keeping a container of vegan Worcestershire Sauce near because it also introduces a pleasant flavor to your appetizing dishes.

Make it spice – I'm unquestionably a big fan of sriracha. See, not every person is into the hot sauce so having a jug of sriracha allows everybody to have their dish to their very own heat inclination. So, I will cook the basic recipe in a generally mellow taste form and then serve hot sauce (or a container of hot sauce) as an afterthought so that people with a spicier flare (ME!) can spruce up the dish as they want.

Become a short order cook – Playing on the thing over this one, I like to purchase things like Lighthouse flavors and herbs that allow me to spruce up my dish just as I like it. For instance, Shawn doesn't really like cilantro all that much. So I can keep cilantro on hand and add as much as I want to my dishes. It's ideal. Same thing with mushrooms. I make a cluster and add them to my recipes so Shawn doesn't need to pick them off his plate.

The best DIY Microwave Popcorn with a recipe for Nooch Popcorn. It's without butter, healthy, reasonable, and OH so tasty! Simply Say CHEESE – You can purchase vegetarian parmesan, or make handcrafted vegan parmesan. I recommend having some on hand to sprinkle over your recipes. Also, dietary yeast drops (now and then alluded to as nooch) is incredible stuff to have around. You can get it in most supermarkets and it's ideal for giving a marginally nutty, gooey flavor to generally bland dishes. I've even added it to my DIY Vegan Cheesy Popcorn! There are also some really extraordinary vegan cheddar items out there. Our top picks are Daiya and Follow Your Heart.

Get Saucy – I love a good sauce. And having a sauce you can serve over your favorite dishes will have a significant effect. I've made a Vegan Queso sauce that can be used over a variety of vegan Mexican dishes. And I made a vegan pesto that I've served over an assortment of pasta dishes. And there's nothing like a good vegan alfredo sauce that can be served with pasta and even pizza!

I trust you enjoyed these Vegan Cooking Tips and Tricks! Discover more vegan cooking recipes on our assets page. Also, if you're interested in what sort of vegan you are (or maybe sometime in the not so distant future), take my 3 Kinds of Vegan Survey!

Chapter 14: Tips for Losing Weight on a Vegan Diet

Up your protein, bring down your soy, and as usual: go for the greens

As indicated by an article published in the Journal of General Internal Medicine, people who follow a vegetarian diet for roughly 18 weeks shed, by and large, four pounds more than those who follow animal-based diets. While this reality is amazing for anyone hoping to get in shape, switching to a plant-based diet and weight loss are not instantly synonymous.

Many people who change to a vegan diet for weight loss reasons often wind up filling the meatless void with a variety of plant-based foods. Fortunately, a vegan diet is far beyond pre-packed foods that simply happen to be fat-free, especially for those hoping to get in shape. By following these six hints, you'll fit into your favorite pair of pants in the blink of an eye, all while doing what is right.

Survey the vegan food pyramid

The foundation of the vegan food pyramid is greens and vegetables followed by fruits. This is a refreshed variant of MyPyramid—the food guide that replaced the Food Guide Pyramid in 2005—which emphasized grains, bread, oat, and pasta as the foundation of a good healthy diet. In spite of the fact that the vegetarian food pyramid fills in as a guide, caloric admission and portion control are key variables for any get-healthy plan.

Eat greens

The versatility of spinach, broccoli, Swiss chard, bok choy, Brussels sprouts, and zucchini makes dark leafy greens a great addition to any meal. These foods are perfect for weight loss because they are the "most supplement thick healthy things" and "are incredibly low in calories and high in fibre," says Lisa Odenweller, CEO of Santa Monica-based super-food bistro, Beaming. The high-fibre content keeps you satisfied for the whole day while helping you avoid unhealthy snacking. Other high-fibre choices include fruits (be aware of the sugar substance) and crude tree nuts (almonds, walnuts, and cashews), which are stuffed with protein and fibre and can help lower cholesterol.

Up your protein

Use of protein-rich food is important in many get-healthy plans because protein fills you up faster; therefore, you need less food to be satisfied. As per Stephanie Gold finger of vegan site Cooking for Luv, proteins are accessible in numerous forms, which makes them helpful to include in meals because they can be eaten raw or quickly cooked. Protein powders are perfect for a snatch and-go breakfast or noontime smoothie, while other plant-based proteins, for example, tempeh, beans, lentils, quinoa, and oats are flexible and can fill in as the primary part of a veggie burrito, salad, or pan-fried food.

Limit Processed Soy

Soy products can be the easiest and most helpful "go-to" things when changing to a vegan diet. Soy isn't really unhealthy, but it is important that consideration is given to the amount of processed food in a meal plan. For example, a tofu scramble for breakfast, soy veggie burger for lunch, and cushion Thai with tofu for dinner is over the top. Rather, pick vegan cheddar made with nuts, a brown bean burger, or a cushion Thai with vegetables and tempeh for whole food modifications of your favorite foods.

Plan Healthy Meals

Meal plan is an imperative part to guarantee appropriate nutrition and weight loss, and, fortunately, grocery stores currently sell pre-packed vegetables that are table-ready in minutes. Instances of fast-and-easy dishes incorporate quinoa bowls with tempeh; a mixed sautéed food mix of broccoli, carrots, and mushrooms; eggplant cutlets with marinara sauce, veggie lover cheddar, and basil; and soba noodles with greens. If these meals are past your extension, meal conveyance administrations, for example, HelloFresh and meal plan administrations, for example, Plate Joy give easy-to-pursue recipes that are pre-amount and dietitian-approved.

Get exercise and remain hydrated

Healthy meals, water, and exercise are key parts of any effective get-healthy plan. People ought to participate in 150 minutes of moderate cardio or 75 minutes of energetic high-impact activity each week, to burn calories and get thinner. High-Intensity Interval Training (HIIT) is a type of cardiovascular interim training that focuses on substituting brief periods of extreme anaerobic exercise with slower recovery periods. To achieve best results, HIIT ought to be done three times per week and combined with running or climbing, says Jorge Cruise, coach, and creator of Tiny and Full. And remember to remain hydrated! Drinking at least 64 ounces of water every day keeps your body clean, which improves wellness and overall health.

Chapter 15: Make a Grocery List

Stay sorted with a basic needs list to avoid buying things you don't really need.

The initial step to gainful shopping for food is making a list of the things you need to purchase. So we have for you today How to Make an Organized Grocery List {Free Printable}.

Going shopping for food without a basic needs list can prompt you to carelessly wander the store without a detailed plan, just to return home with a bunch of things you don't need and without those that you do. Having a basic supply list has numerous advantages like keeping you on the healthy track and avoiding extra outings to the store.

Making a basic needs list doesn't have to be difficult or tedious. Truth be told, it tends to be easy and fun, especially when you have a free printable to use.

Feeling sorted out in any aspect of your life removes that dreadful pressure factor.

Use your list of weekly meals.
Make a list of foods and refreshments you need to buy to make the meals in your weekly plan. Remember to incorporate foods like fruits, vegetables, and milk that probably won't be included in a recipe but are basics for healthy eating.

Sort out your list.
Make shopping fast and easy by sorting out your list into different areas or food groups. For a free format, attempt the Create a Grocery Game Plan: Grocery List.

Include foods as you go.
Keep a continuous staple list in your kitchen or on a free portable application, and include things as you run out. Some versatile applications allow you to match up staple records with others in your household.

Follow These Steps to Make an Organized Grocery List

Stage 1: Have a Running List
Have a "to purchase" list somewhere in your home. Use this running list to monitor things that you have run out or are close to running out and need to be replaced.

Stage 2: Meal Plan
Meal planning is the most ideal approach to guarantee that you are just purchasing things that you require, sticking to your spending plan and remaining sorted out.

Stage 3: Take Inventory Of Staple Foods
The initial step to making a basic needs list is to check your storeroom and fridge and take stock of any staple foods that need replacing. Eggs, Milk, Butter, Granola Bars and any canned products you use daily should be a need.

Stage 4: Look Up Coupons
Look into different coupons and specials that are accessible to you before closing your list. In addition, if you discover an order on something that you normally run out of constantly, you can stock up and set aside some money.

Stage 5: Print A Grocery List Printable
We have a FREE online staple list printable to enable you to deal with your basic needs list. Utilizing our printable can help you easily master your basic need list in a brisk and

efficient way, with a beautiful and all around arranged layout.

Stage 6: Organize By Aisle
To make your shopping trip less tedious and work concentrated, sort out your list as indicated by the walkways in your supermarket. If you isolate your list into areas, it's a lot easier to guarantee that nothing goes neglected. This is the reason using our free printable is useful as it's as of now, separated into perfect segments.

Stage 7: Specify Quantity
The amount of one thing is imperative when making your list. It is great to know the amount of a thing you need to get ahead of time.

Stage 8: Check Your List
Try to go over your list and make any last minute alterations before you leave for the store. If necessary, prepare a duplicate list.

Stage 9: Don't Leave It

Try not to leave your list on the counter! Ensure that you put it somewhere you won't forget before you leave for your shopping trip.

There are many other approaches to guarantee that your Grocery list is efficient. Make a point to monitor things you run out of regularly, look into coupons and use our Grocery List Printable whenever possible.

Perhaps you're a ninja in the kitchen. Perhaps you're simply beginning your cooking experience. In any case, these tips and tricks from gourmet experts and food aces can help you spend less energy sweating over an oven and more time getting a charge out of the foods of your work.

We tossed a wide net asking food specialists to include their most useful tips. You definitely know a large number of these, but out and out the tips structure is a manual for wasting less time in the kitchen.

The Basics

Many of the gourmet specialists' tips were pretty basics but require rehashing.

1. Read recipes in full before you begin cooking. It's an easy decision, but when you're in the race to eat cooked food or feel you know what you're doing, you may disregard this basic initial step. Emilie Bousquet-Walshe, Chef de Cuisine of Go Burger Bar and Grill, says:

The most efficient tool is following recipes to their fullest before beginning, regardless of whether at home or at work. That way you have sufficient energy to begin and some time to complete certain directions, while others are underway. For instance, one of our leaders is in culinary school and asked me to assist her with a cake. She began by taking out all the ingredients and halfway through, I stopped her and advised her to read the directions first. The initial step was to isolate the eggs and keep the egg whites at room temp for 30 minutes. By not reading that, she would have wasted 30 minutes of prep.

2. Use the correct tools. Michelle Girasole, advertising executive for Chef Jamie Oliver, shares this tip:

Get a good set of knives, and figure out how to chop appropriately. A very sharp, adjusted knife set ought to be included in a gourmet specialist's list (8" cutting edge), a small paring knife, and a serrated knife for cakes and breads. This trio will make cleaving easier and more secure, and save time in the kitchen.

3. Pick in-season ingredients. A few culinary specialists rehashed the tip to purchase in-season produce and meats. Not only will this save you money, but you also don't need to do as much with the food to get the best flavors. Gourmet specialist Gregory Gourdet of Departure Restaurant + Lounge in Portland says:

Continuously work with too seasonal ingredients for greatest flavor, you should do less to them to make them taste delicious. This will save you time and calories!

4. Try not to strip all produce. Chef Gregory proceeds:

Eat the skin! All fruits and vegetables have supplement and fibre rich skin, so if you have delicate products don't try stripping. Simply ensure it is washed well. Carrots, sweet potatoes, and beets all roast up amazing skin on.

5. Keep in mind the "mise en place"...for a few recipes. Prep your ingredients before you start and you can maintain a strategic distance from recipe disasters (and time-wasting revisions). Regardless of whether you use small dishes on your counter, a solitary bowl, or a biscuit tin for your mise en place, it often—but not usually—pays to get all of your ingredients prepared in the beginning.

Shelley Young, Chef and Owner of The Chopping Block in Chicago, prompts:

It's all about "mise en place", which is French for "together in place". Regularly, have all of your ingredients available and prepared to go before you begin cooking. For certain recipes where the dish is cooked in all respects rapidly, for example, sautéed food or Chicken Picatta, you ought to have all of your ingredients sliced and prepared ahead of time before you begin to cook. For different dishes, for example, soup which cooks longer, you can spare time by doing the prep function as you cook as opposed to having everything sliced and prepared to go ahead of time.

6. Prep your container. In addition to preparing ingredients, prepare your container

too. Dave Feller, author, and CEO of Yummly, says:

Begin with HOT dish: Instead of putting a cool dish on the oven, at that point including oil, turning on the head and wait for it to get warm, begin with an empty skillet on the oven. It will get hotter as you prep your ingredients, making it the ideal temperature for your food (and cooks faster!)

David Craine, Executive Chef of BLT Bar and Grill in New York City concurs:

Put the container you plan on utilizing in a preheating oven. That way, they'll be hot when you're prepared to use them.

7. Cook once, get ready many times. And make extra. This is a procedure I've been attempting to use because it's more proficient to make two-for-one meals. Beth Bader, the creator of The Cleaner Plate Club, offers many extraordinary tips:

- a) Cook once, plan numerous ways. Long-cook things like roast chicken are for a considerable length of time, but left-over chicken can make a snappy stew with canned beans, chicken serving of mixed greens or chicken for plates of mixed greens, quesadillas and other easy, fast weeknight meals. Roast two chickens in that oven when you have sufficient energy! Serve one, cut and use the scraps for easy weeknight meals and lunches. In addition, the two carcasses will give you a chance to make double the stock for soups in one go as well!

b) Cook double batches of soups, bean stews, even spaghetti sauce and freeze half for a bustling week. After a couple of times of this, you have an entire week's meals prepared to defrost in the microwave and heat for the evenings when you don't have room schedule-wise to cook or when you are too occupied to do the week's cooking throughout the end of the week!

Use weekend family time to get help preparing extensive meals for the week. By making these meals on Saturday and Sunday, you ought to have scraps to interchange Monday-Wednesday. A snappy meal on Thursday like flame-broiled cheddar and soup (from your fridge stash) and make-your-very own pizza and salad night on Fridays for entertainment only and you have real food on the table without cooking each night!

Jeff Anderson, Executive Chef for Safeway Culinary Kitchens, Recommends you toss in an additional roast when making a pork midsection, pot roast, or other things—so you'll have extra to cut into sandwiches and different meals.

Remember this applies to desserts as well. Laura Forer of Waltzing Matilda's Bakery in New York stated:

Want new cookies but would prefer not to bake up an entire batch? Next time you are making cookies, make a double clump. While your cookies are baking, take the additional batter and scoop it out onto a sheet skillet fixed with parchment paper. Pop the skillet in the fridge for around 30 minutes. When frozen, put the unbaked cookies in a sack and freeze until you're prepared to use them. You can then make small bunches of newly baked cookies whenever!

8. Spare even the smallest of meals. Little portions of ingredients can be transformed into "enhance bombs" for your next meals, says Gio Bellino of, well, Flavor Bombs:

Get in the habit of freezing bits of meals! What I mean by that is saving small amounts of that delicious sauce on your meatloaf, save the chicken fat you skim from your soup, save a portion of that bacon grease (especially the maple enhanced mmmm), save a portion of that rub, marinade, herb mix. Saving small amounts of stuffing or vegetables will provide you with a flavorful mixture to either puree for a sauce or reuse as a breading. Having these components in your fridge will make cooking future dishes a snap. You begin trying different things with mixing flavors, you have starters on hand to make another dish from flavors you now love.

Once you have this tendency, you build up a store of ingredients in your fridge that spare you time and money. You are basically making your own "flavor bombs".

Stacey Strout Stabenow, Organizer of No More 'to go' Weekly Meal Plan, has similar ideas:

If a recipe requires dicing small amounts of vegetables like onion or chime peppers, feel free to dice the entire thing. Store the rest in a resalable sack in the fridge; huge help for future recipes.

When using halfway jars of things like creamed corn or stews in adobo, name and store the rest of resealable bags.

The same goes for new herbs. If you have more than you need, basically freeze the rest in ice block plate. Spot the herbs in the plate, load up with water and freeze. When frozen, exchange to resealable bags. To defrost, just flush in heated water, pat dry, and use as if they were new.

9. Clean as you go. Since tidying up is one of the most terrible parts of cooking, David Lebovitz's most beloved kitchen tip ever is also one of my top picks:

Essentially fill the sink with warm, soapy water, and as you finish with dishes, slide them into the water. Afterward, they'll be easier to clean after a relaxed drenching, and you simply rub or scour them with a wipe and pile them up in the dishwasher. Or on the other hand, finish washing by hand.

10. Cook more "one pot" meals. Beth Moncel tells The Kitchen that one pot meals are easy to make, and result in fewer dirty dishes, and usually freeze and warm great.

11. Prep for the week. Regardless of whether you spend an entire day for clump cooking or only one hour throughout the end of the week, preparing your vegetables can spare you time during the more hectic weeks' of work. First, slash all your onions, haul out your food processor to grind carrots and cabbage, and so forth., and then pack the prepared veggies up. This spares time as well as obviously makes it more likely that you'll cook during the week. We prescribe that people use this opportunity to perform various tasks - investing energy with a relative or making up for lost time with their beloved podcast.

More Specific Tips

Some of the tips we got was specific to certain kinds of foods but still worth adding to your stockpile of cooking tricks.

12. Push the roasting temperature. You don't need to rely upon a recipe's cooking temperature all of the time.

Roast at a higher temperature. Your oven has temperatures other than 350. A few things, for example, roasted vegetables, fish, and baked grains, actually cook better at higher temperatures. And the higher temperatures cook them faster. For instance, you can bake shrimp at 450 and they're done in 5 minutes. If you roast veggies at 400 versus 350, you can shave 15-20 minutes off their cooking time.

13. Saute vegetables before including stock or water. Mihaela Lica Butler, the creator of Garden Super Hero Tales, offers this tip for making soup:

For vegetable soups, sauté the veggies before you add the stock or on the other hand, the water. This strategy improves the taste by allowing the flavors to mix and decreases cooking time by 5 to 10 minutes.

14. Mash parmesan cheddar at room temperature. The cheddar is milder which makes it easier to grind, and more averse to cause a cut on the grater, exhorts Chef Mirko Paderno, Executive Chef at Oliverio. He also offers this other efficient tip:

15. Cook dried beans in mineral water. Obviously, the additional components in the water help the beans cook faster.

16. Beat egg whites before the yolks. Dancing Matilda's bakery also says:

If a recipe, for example, whip cake or feathery omelets—calls for beating yolks and whites separately, beat the whites first. That way, you don't need to wash the mixers in between. (If you beat the yolks first, the lingering yolk may cause the whites not to increase in volume as easily.) Then give the whites a snappy whip when you're prepared to use them to re-swell them. Now, any leftover on the blenders won't have any kind of effect.

17. Roast beets whole. Whoopee, no stripping! Recipe engineer Pamela Braun

MyMansBelly.com says:

A big-deal saver in the kitchen is roasting beets whole. Wrap the beets in foil with a touch of coarse salt and olive oil. Throw them in the oven to roast. When they're set, the skins will slip off easily. This saves loads of time stripping and shields your hands from getting recolored.

18. Time to what extent it takes to warm oil in a container (and then use a clock going ahead). Beauty Young tells The Kitchen:

Use a clock to preheat the wok. My wok preheats in 1 minute on my gas oven and to spare testing the wok's heat, I simply set my clock.

She also offers this performing multiple tasks tip:

19. Use remaining heated water to completely wipe germs. "After boiling water for some tea, I pour the rest of the water from the pot over the dish wipe."

20. Skip caramelizing meat before adding to your slow cooker by "using a little soy sauce and tomato paste (mystery weapons) to add the same great depth of flavor," as indicated by America's Test Kitchen/The Blade.

Chapter 16: How to make boring food tasty with ingredients

If you're preparing, cooking, or plating and feel that your food doesn't display the wow factor you wish it would, most of the time, simply switching up the ingredients and garnishes puts a tremendous twist to a generally normal (otherwise known as, exhausting) dish.

Basically Citrus
Citrus fruits can literally turn into your best kitchen sous chef expert and can be included into pretty much everything. There's an overall variety of ways to use citrus and include a bit, or a lot, of get-up-and-go to your favorite nom-ables.

Everyone knows that citrus has vitamin C, but did you know that these fruits have a significant amount of fibre as well? Fibre has been known to help overall absorption as well as controlling glucose levels.

Mesh skins of orange, lime, or grapefruit for pizzazz and add it to anything you're cooking—

sweet and appetizing. Get-up-and-go includes acidity and lights up both sweet and appetizing flavors. Extra points if you grind some on the highest part of your beloved pastry or mix to make seasoned sugars. Goodness me, extravagant!

Press lemon into pretty much any saucy dish and its taste will be greatly improved. Everything from marinara and alfredo sauce to bean stew, stews, and soups are kicked up with a bit of harsh. Please, don't stop me.

Slammin' Herbs
Use herbs and flavors in ways that you may have never thought of. Mysterious inventions can often happen while saying to yourself "what might happen if I added some herbal punch to that?"

Yellow curry powder is an incredibly versatile seasoning. Take a stab at adding a portion of that decency into mashed potatoes or even plain old rice for an instant picker-upper. I love including curried rice into tacos or making a rice and bean stuffing for veggies like squash or ringer peppers. The turmeric in curry has been said to be used as a mitigating which assists with aching joint and muscle pains, making it one of nature's actual superfoods.

Everybody cherishes cinnamon, but for reasons unknown, we, for the most part, observe it in sweet dessert dishes. Cinnamon is known to enable our bodies to regulate insulin which controls our glucose, making it one more reason to add to veggie or meat stews and rubs for chicken, pork or hamburger.

Incredible Gains with Grains
Tired of plain rice? It occurs. Mix up the mealtime standard with whole grains that include naturalness and health benefits that turn bland to grand.

Quinoa is naturally gluten-free, stuffed with huge amounts of iron, and makes an insane good breakfast food. If you're trapped in an endless cycle of eating oats or oat for breakfast most days, quinoa is easy to make in large batches and stays in the fridge for later days. Add some cinnamon, sugar, and foods grown from the ground too will end up turning into a quinoa ruler.

Lentils can be used practically anywhere that you would normally use beans. They're my go-to when food is making me yawn on account of their complex carbs and they've been said to increase energy levels. How about we move! They work incredibly in soups, burritos, and even in plates of mixed greens.

Go Flippin' Nuts
Regardless of whether your paleo, vegetarian, low-fat, high-fat, carb viewing or out and out ravenous, nuts and seeds are each diet companion on account of the jam stuffed protein in every little chunk.

Include nuts and seeds as toppers to a salad or include it into your pan-fried food. Sweet and salty flavors quite often mix well together.

Include sunflower seed butter as an alternative to nutty spread. Much as it is America's most loved topping, this butter is extraordinary on hotcakes, in a smoothie, or even when added to pan-fried food to make a tasty "nut sauce." Sunflower seeds have huge amounts of vitamin E and are said to keep your skin super healthy. Butter up, buttercup.

Drop some hemp hearts over your hummus dunk or sprinkle it in with your chocolate spread (chocolate and banana sandwiches are fantastic!). This will include a one of a kind nutty flavor and hemp hearts contain 10 grams of protein for every 2 tablespoons! Which is actually equivalent to 2 medium sized eggs. Your friends will believe you're a culinary virtuoso.

Productive Success
Vegetables may appear like an easy choice, but you can imagine (signal your best insane lab rat evil laugh) some unquestionably imaginative and lovely darn great sides with fruits that will leave visitors asking for the recipe.

Cut up some mango or nectarines and include it into your next salsa. Vegetable salsas are easy to make and you don't need a food processor (thick salsa is impressive!). This sweet, salty, and fiery mixture is scrumptious with chips but really stands out when bested on pork, chicken, or as an essential topper for Mexican food.

Mangoes are very enzymatic and have huge amounts of acidic chemicals that support unrelated foods and can help clear stomach related problems. They carry out double responsibility outwardly too as a skin chemical.

Raspberries, strawberries, blackberries, and apples are a cool way to keep plates of mixed greens poppin' as a customary side dish or for a primary for those of us who are attempting to eat somewhat healthier. Furthermore, the best part is no cooking is involved—simply thud them directly on top and voila!

Extra Points! Chewing and biting the skin on apples has been said to help advance healthy teeth as well as keep them white.

Chapter 17: Instructions to Make Boring Food Taste Amazing

Currently, this is the means by which to cook cauliflower, Brussels sprouts, tilapia, and other potentially ho-murmur meal staples.

Transform Cauliflower into Steak
The old way: Trim off and dispose of the stems; roast or heat up the florets.

The new way: Sear it and bake it—like you would do a rib eye—which makes the outside fresh and inside delicate. Reward: You don't throw anything out. Cut the whole head into inch-thick cuts, framing cauliflower "steaks." Season with salt and pepper, and cook in a couple of tablespoons of vegetable oil until brown, around three minutes for each side. Finish in a 350-degree oven, cooking for 10 minutes or until delicate.

Carry Tilapia to the Tropics
The old way: Olive oil, garlic, lemon, sear, yawn.

The new way: Pair the fish (which broadly—or notoriously, contingent upon how much you like seafood—doesn't taste like fish) with intense flavors. Our most recent go-to: Puree some mango pieces, a dash of coconut milk and much smaller dashes of fish sauce and bean stew powder; at that point, pour the sauce over the seared filet.

Purchase the Right Brussels Sprouts
The old way: Sauté them with bacon or pancetta.

The new way: Go ahead and cook these vegetables with your preferred smoked meat, but use infant Brussels sprouts. Since a vegetable's flavor will, in general, intensify as the plant develops, more youthful forms frequently taste less unpleasant and are increasingly delicate (in this way needing less cooking). Melissa's sells baby sprouts in slick clamshell bundles (check Melissas.com to discover a store close you).

Cook Brown Rice Without Water
The old way: Simmer the rice in a pot with the cover firmly fixed.

The new way: Precook the rice to include a toasty flavor and then finish it in a similar sauté container. Broil the uncooked grains with a teaspoon or two of olive oil. A couple of minutes later, add a clove of minced garlic. When the dish becomes aromatic, blend in chicken stock (as much as you would have used water). Stew until the rice is cooked.

Fresh Up Baby New Potatoes
The old way: Boil and throw in vinaigrette.

The new way: Cook scoured potatoes in boiling water, but only for 15 minutes, until they're sufficiently delicate that, when they've cooled a bit, you can smash them marginally with the base of your clench hand (or the end of a durable juice glass). Throw them in a roasting dish with a covering of olive oil and salt; and roast at 400 degrees until the smashed edges of the potatoes start to appear dark colored and fresh. Add minced garlic and whatever chopped herbs you'd like (mint, basil, rosemary, thyme); serve.

Chapter 18: Preventing Foodborne Illnesses

Food-handling and Storage Procedures

Proper food handling can prevent most foodborne diseases. For pathogens to develop in food, certain conditions must be present. By controlling the soil conditions, regardless of whether potentially harmful bacteria are available in the raw food, they most certainly won't survive, grow, and multiply, causing sickness.

There are six factors that influence bacterial development, which can be alluded to by the memory aide FATTOM:

- Food
- Acid
- Temperature
- Time
- Oxygen
- Moisture

Every one of these variables contributes to bacterial development in the following ways:

- Food: Bacteria need food to survive. Therefore, sodden, protein-rich foods are great potential wellsprings of bacterial development.
- Acid: Bacteria don't develop in acidic conditions. This is the reason acidic foods like lemon juice and vinegar don't bolster the development of bacteria and can be used as additives
- Temperature: Most bacteria will develop quickly between 4°C and 60°C (40°F and 140°F). This is alluded to as the risk zone (see the area underneath for more data on the peril zone).
- Time: Bacteria need time to multiply. When small quantities of bacteria are present, the hazard is usually low, but over time, the right conditions will allow the bacteria to multiply and increase the danger of sullying.
- Oxygen: There are two types of bacteria. High-impact bacteria which need oxygen to grow, so won't multiply without oxygen, for example, a vacuum-bundled holder. Anaerobic bacteria will just develop sans oxygen. Food that has been inappropriately prepared and then stored at room temperature can be in danger from anaerobic bacteria. A

typical precedent is a product containing harmful Clostridium botulinum (botulism-causing) bacteria that has been inappropriately prepared during canning and then is consumed without further cooking or warming.

➢ Moisture: Bacteria need dampness to survive and will develop quickly in wet foods. This is the reason dry and salted foods are at lower risk of being dangerous.

Identifying Potentially Hazardous Foods (PHFs)

Foods that have these FATTOM conditions are viewed as potentially harmful foods (PHFs). PHFs are those foods that are viewed as short-lived. That is, they will spoil or "turn sour" if left at room temperature. PHFs are foods that help the development or survival of disease-causing bacteria (pathogens) or foods that might be tainted by pathogens.

Generally, a food is a PHF if it is:

➢ Of animal source, for example, meat, milk, eggs, fish, shellfish, poultry (or if it contains any of these items)

- Of plant source (vegetables, beans, fruits, and so forth.) that has been heat-treated or cooked
- Any of the raw sprouts (bean, horse feed, radish, and so forth.)
- Any cooked starch (rice, pasta, and so on.)
- Any sort of soya protein (soya milk, tofu, and so on.)

Table identifies normal foods as either PHF or non-PHF.

PHF	Non-PHF
Chicken, beef, pork, and other meats	Beef jerky
Pastries filled with meat, cheese, or cream	Bread
Cooked rice	Uncooked rice

Fried onions	Raw onions
Opened cans of meat, vegetables, etc.	Unopened cans of meat, vegetables, etc. (as long as they are not marked with "Keep Refrigerated")
Tofu	Uncooked beans
Coffee creamers	Cooking oil
Fresh garlic in oil	Fresh garlic
Fresh or cooked eggs	Powdered eggs
Gravy	Flour

Dry soup mix with water added	Dry soup mix

Table: Basic PHF and non-PHFs

The Danger Zone

The most imperative elements to think about when handling food properly is temperature. Table 3 shows the temperatures to know about when handling food.

Celsius	Fahrenheit	
100°	212°	Water boils
60°	140°	Most pathogenic bacteria are destroyed. Keep hot foods above this temperature.

20°	68°	Food must be cooled from 60°C to 20°C (140°F to 68°F) within two hours or less
4°	40°	Food must be cooled from 20°C to 4°C (68°F to 40°F) within four hours or less
0°	32°	Water freezes
−18°	0°	Frozen food must be stored at −18°C (0°F) or below

Table: Vital temperatures to recall

The scope of temperature from 4°C and 60°C (40°F and 140°F) is known as the threat zone, or the range at which most pathogenic bacteria will develop and duplicate.

Time-temperature Control of PHFs

Pathogen development is constrained by a period temperature relationship. To kill small scale living beings, food must be kept at an adequate temperature for an adequate time. Cooking is a programmed procedure in which a sequence of persistent temperature blends can be equally successful. For instance, when cooking a meat roast, the microbial lethality accomplished at 121 minutes after it has achieved an inner temperature of 54°C (130°F) is equivalent to if it were cooked for 3 minutes after it had achieved 63°C (145°F).

The table below demonstrates the base time-temperature necessities to safeguard food. (Other time-temperature regimens may be reasonable if it very well may be illustrated, with scientific information that the routine results in a preserved food.)

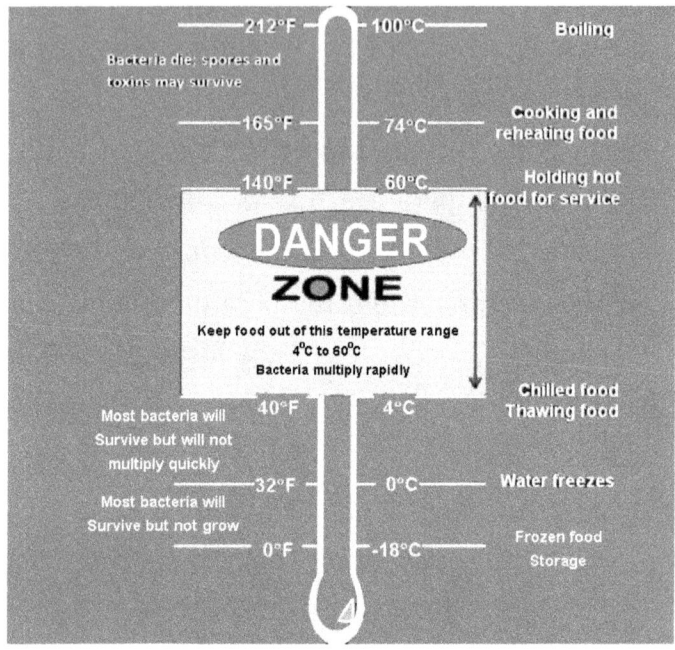

Figure: Threat Zone Chart, Used with consent from BC Center for Disease Control (BCCDC)

Critical control point	Temperature
Refrigeration	
Cold food storage: all foods	4°C (40°F) or less
Freezing	
Frozen food storage – all foods	–18°C (0°F) or less
Parasite reduction in fish intended to be served raw, such as sushi and sashimi **Raw fish**	–20°C (–4°F) for 7 days or, –35°C (–31°F) in a blast freezer for 15 hours
Cooking	
Food mixtures containing poultry, eggs, meat, fish, or other potentially hazardous foods	Internal temperature of 74°C (165°F) for at least 15 seconds
Rare roast beef	Internal temperature of 54°C to 60°C (130°F to 140°F)

Medium roast beef	Internal temperature of 60°C to 65°C (140°F to 150°F)
Pork, lamb, veal, beef (medium-well)	Internal temperature of 65°C to 69°C (150°F to 158°F)
Pork, lamb, veal, beef (well done)	Internal temperature of 71°C (160°F)
Poultry	Internal temperature of 74°C (165°F) for 15 seconds
Stuffing in poultry	74°C (165°F)
Ground meat[1]	70°C (158°F)
Eggs[2]	63°C (145°F) for 15 seconds
Fish[3]	70°C (158°F)
Holding, cooling, and reheating	
Holding hot foods	60°C (140°F)
Cooling	60°C to 20°C (140°F to 68°F) within 2 hours and 20°C to 4°C (68°F to 40°F) within 4 hours

Reheating	74°C (165°F) for at least 15 seconds

Table: Temperature control for PHFs

Learn the labels

- Do not eat or taste food from jars that lump or spill or that have a sticky buildup or a strange smell. The food could be debased.
- Read food packaging marks for directions on the most proficient method to store foods after opening and for expiry dates.
- Note the different kinds of termination language. FSIS gives a list of what to search for:
- A "Sell-by" date advises the store to what extent to display the item available to be purchased. Purchase the item before the date expires.
- A "Best if used by" (or "Before") date is suggested for best flavor or quality.
- A "Use-by" date is the last date prescribed to use the item at pinnacle quality. The date has been controlled by the maker.

Patricia Buck, executive of Outreach and Education at the Center for Foodborne Illness Research and Prevention, prescribes the accompanying shopping tips:

- Ensure beyond reasonable doubt that the product isn't damaged because pathogens are bound to develop on damaged areas.
- Be mindful of organism developing on the product because spores could be inside it.
- Check for creepy crawlies on produce.
- Raw meat, poultry, and fish can be contaminated with bacteria, so it is ideal to put the item in a sack to decrease cross-sullying with other basic supply things.
- If your neighborhood food merchant does not keep bags at the meat counter, propose it.
- Review CFI's Six Safe Food Practices for extra tips.

Dangerous foods

It's imperative to remember that certain foods regularly sold in stores or ranchers markets are not suitable for customers who are pregnant, old, young or who have a weak immune system.

Washington State University's School of Food Science prescribes the following safeguards for eating potentially harmful foods:

- ➢ Drink just pasteurized milk and fruits juices.
- ➢ Use water from a sheltered water supply for drinking and food preparation.
- ➢ Avoid eating raw sprouts.
- ➢ Avoid eating raw or undercooked seafood.
- ➢ Avoid eating foods containing raw eggs; use pasteurized eggs or egg products in uncooked foods containing eggs.
- ➢ Use cheddar and yogurt prepared using pasteurized milk.

Obtain shellfish from sources that are affirmed by the government or State food health organizations.

If you're pregnant, older or have a compromised immune system:

- ➢ Avoid mild cheeses, cold smoked fish, or cold shop plates of mixed greens.

> Avoid sausage and lunch meats that have not been warmed to steaming hot or 165 degrees.

Ohio State University's Agricultural Research and Development Center records the following as dangerous foods for kids:

> - Raw (unpasteurized) dairy products, for example, milk, cheddar, and yogurt
> - Unpasteurized fruits juices
> - Raw sprouts
> - Undercooked meat, for example, ground hamburger
> - Raw eggs, like those found in cookie batter

Food readiness

Avoid contamination from food handlers, different foods, and the surrounding conditions.

Defrosting, cooking and chilling

> - Proper temperature is essential to protect food.
> - Buy a food thermometer to guarantee you are cooking raw meats and eggs to appropriate temperatures.

- Store food immediately in a fridge at 40 F. Try not to over-burden fridges as that may keep cool air from flowing.
- Defrost food from the fridge, in cold water or in the microwave.

Chapter 19: Meal plan for 6 weeks

When you realize it's time to clean up your diet, nixing takeout and packaged comfort foods is need number one. Commercially prepared meals will, in general, be stuffed with shrouded sugar, sodium, and unhealthy fats, and portions are often far greater than what you'd normally serve yourself. That is the reason scientific research has proved that cooking at home as often as possible is associated with a healthier diet, paying little heed to whether somebody's endeavoring to get in shape.

Thing is, planning nutritious meals is difficult. I'm an enrolled dietitian, and one of the most well-known complaints I get from my customers is that they simply don't have sufficient energy to cook each and every night of the week. And I totally get it—you presumably wear a great deal many hats (parent, spouse, friend, guardian, supervisor), and "gourmet specialist" isn't one of them.

That is the reason I am collaborating with Prevention and Delish on the Meal Prep Reset.

With this arrangement, I'll be providing you with a month of healthy meal prep recipes, including breakfasts, lunches, dinners, and snacks.

What is meal preparing, exactly?

It's so simple. "Meal prep recipes" are simply recipes intended to be set aside a few minutes in one main batch. You cook once and then have healthy breakfasts, lunches, and dinners prepared for nearly the whole week. Read more about health advantages, techniques, and strategizing your menu in my inside and out guide on the most proficient method to meal prep.

Who says waffles are just for the end of the week? Make these low-carb waffles on Sunday, store them in the refrigerator, and then eventually pop them in the toaster to warm up.

How the Meal Prep Reset functions?

The recipes below are intended to be prepared on Sunday and then eaten Monday through Thursday, the busiest part of the week. Do your shopping on Saturday or early Sunday, and then spend Sunday afternoon or night cooking and packing up your food (plan on 1 to 2 hours in the kitchen). These recipes will give you four servings each.

But imagine a scenario where you would prefer not to prepare ALL of your meals. You don't need to! This plan is totally adaptable based upon your needs and objectives. A number of my customers have no issue preparing breakfast each morning, but battle with lunch and dinner; others are stars at putting together a lunch, but can't shake the drive-through breakfast sandwich propensity.

Is this meal prep plan for weight loss?

I structured the Meal Prep Reset to enable you to accomplish three objectives:

- ➤ Load your diet with lean protein, healthy carbs and fats, and savvy snacks, while taking out processed junk.
- ➤ Nix your takeout propensity.
- ➤ Learn new healthy cooking methods, like foil bundle recipes, stuffed baked potatoes, noodles, overnight oats, and many more.

As you can see, getting in shape isn't on this list. All things considered, if you once in a while cook now and your present diet comprises of a ton of fast food, frozen meals, and packaged snacks, following this plan may in truth help you drop a couple of pounds. By cooking your own meals, you'll simply start expending less sugar, salt, and unhealthy fats, which may thus enable you to cut excess calories.

Meal prep compartments and other tools you'll need for the Meal Prep Reset

Meal preparing is tied in with saving time—and having the correct kitchen tools and meal prep compartments prepared to go is key to doing that. Try not to stress, there's no need to go out and purchase a huge amount of new stuff. Add these extras to the basics you likely now have on hand (like pots and containers, mixing bowls, a sharp knife, and a strong cutting board), and you'll have all that you need to meal prep like a genius.

Week 1 Breakfast: Magic Low-Carb Waffles

Keto waffles are my number one winning breakfast that has prevailed upon some high-carb sweethearts! Keep any extras and use them as sweet sandwich bread for school lunches. Place cream cheddar and berries inside for a yummy lunch box.

Prep Time: 10 mins, Cook Time: 20 mins, Total Time: 30 mins, Serves: 4

Ingredients

> 5 eggs - medium separated
>
> 4 tbsp coconut flour
>
> 4 tbsp granulated sweetener of choice or more, to taste
>
> 1 tsp baking powder
>
> 2 tsp vanilla
>
> 3 tbsp full-fat milk or cream
>
> 125 g butter melted

Directions

> First bowl.

Whisk the egg whites until firm and structure stiff pinnacles.

Second bowl

Mix the egg yolks, coconut flour, sugar, and heating powder.

Add the softened butter slowly, mixing to guarantee a smooth consistency.

Add the milk and vanilla, mix well.

Gently overlap spoons of the whisked egg whites into the yolk mixture. Try to keep as a significant part of the air and fleeciness as conceivable.

Sufficiently place the waffle mixture into the warm waffle maker to make one waffle. Cook until brilliant.

Repeat until all the mixture has been used.

Week 1 Lunch: Spicey Lime Shrimp and Avocado Salad

Lime juice and cilantro are the key ingredients to making this delicious, healthy salad you'll want to make all through spring. Made with cooked stripped shrimp and the freshest ingredients – avocados, tomatoes, red onion, cilantro, and chopped jalapeño mixed with some crisply crushed lime juice and a pinch of olive oil.

Prep Time: 20 mins, Cook Time: 20 mins, Total Time: 40 mins, Serves: 4

Ingredients

1/4 cup chopped red onion

2 limes, juice of

1 tsp olive oil

1/4 tsp kosher salt, black pepper to taste

1 lb jumbo cooked, peeled shrimp, chopped*

1 medium tomato, diced

1 medium Hass avocado, diced (about 5 oz)

1 jalapeno, seeds removed, diced fine

1 tbsp chopped cilantro

Directions

In a small bowl combine red onion, lime juice, olive oil, salt, and pepper. Give them a chance to marinate for like 5 minutes to soften the type of onion.

In a large bowl mix chopped shrimp, avocado, tomato, jalapeño.

Combine all the ingredients together, including cilantro and delicately mix. Add salt and pepper to taste.

Week 1 Snack: Sweet 'N Salty Chocolate Bark

Prep Time: 15 mins, Cook Time: 25 mins, Total Time: 40 mins, Serves: 4

Ingredients

> 2 (12-oz.) bags of dark chocolate chips, melted
>
> 1/2 c. salted pretzels, roughly chopped
>
> 1/4 c. dried cherries
>
> 1/4 c. unsweetened coconut flakes
>
> 1/4 c. unsalted pistachios, roughly chopped
>
> Flaky sea salt

Directions

Prepare a baking sheet with parchment paper. Pour 33% of the dissolved dull chocolate onto the baking sheet and use a counterbalance spatula to spread into an even layer, 1/8" thick.

Evenly sprinkle with a large portion of the pretzels, fruits, coconut, and pistachios.

Pour over staying liquefied dull chocolate and spread to equally cover ingredients.

Evenly sprinkle with residual pretzels, fruits, coconut, and pistachios. Trimming with flaky ocean salt.

Let it cool until set, 60 minutes, at that point break into pieces. Store back in a resealable container until ready to eat.

Week 1 Dinner: Zoodle Ramen

Prep Time: 25 mins, Cook Time: 15 mins, Total Time: 40 mins, Serves: 4

Ingredients

    2 tablespoons vegetable oil

    5 ounces sliced shiitake mushrooms (about 2 cups)

2 cups shredded napa cabbage

2 teaspoons peeled grated ginger root

2 cloves garlic, minced

1 tablespoon white or yellow miso (soybean paste)

1 tablespoon reduced sodium soy sauce

4 cups Swanson® Certified Organic Vegetable Broth or Swanson® Vegetable Broth

6 cups spiralized zucchini noodles (about 14 ounces)

4 green onion, chopped (about 1/4 cup)

¼ cup shredded red cabbage

4 peeled hard-boiled egg, cut in half

Directions

Heat a large portion of the oil in a 12-inch skillet over medium-high heat. Add the mushrooms and napa cabbage and cook for 5 minutes, mixing occasionally. Remove the mushroom mixture from the skillet.

Heat the rest of the oil in the skillet. Add the ginger and garlic and cook and mix for 30 seconds. Mix in the miso, soy sauce, and stock and heat to a boil. Add the zucchini noodles and cook for 2 minutes or until the zucchini noodles are delicate. Season to taste.

Carefully transfer the zucchini noodles to four dishes. Divide the mushroom mixture and the stock mixture among the dishes. Sprinkle with the green onions and red cabbage and top each with 1 egg.

Week 2 Breakfast: Best-Ever Egg Muffins

Prep Time: 15 mins, Cook Time: 20 mins, Total Time: 35 mins, Serves: 12

Ingredients

BASE:

12 large eggs

2 tablespoons finely chopped onion, (red, white or yellow/brown)

Salt and pepper, to taste

TOMATO SPINACH MOZZARELLA:

1/4 cup fresh spinach, roughly chopped

8 grape or cherry tomatoes, halved

1/4 cup shredded mozzarella cheese

Directions

Preheat oven to 350°F | 180°C. Gently drizzle a 12-container limit biscuit tin with nonstick oil splash.

In a large bowl, whisk together the eggs and onion. Season with salt and pepper, to taste.

Add egg mixture all the way up into the greased biscuit tin.

Divide the three fixing mixes into 4 biscuit glasses each.

Bake for 20 minutes.

Serve OR store in a water/air proof container in the fridge for as long as 4 days and warm when ready to serve.

Enjoy!

Prep Time: 20 mins, Cook Time: 20 mins, Total Time: 40 mins, Serves: 4

Ingredients

4 tbsp. hummus

1 medium cucumber, peeled and sliced into matchsticks

2 medium carrots, peeled and sliced into matchsticks

1 c. shredded purple cabbage

2 avocados, pitted and sliced

3 oz. shredded chicken or sautéed tofu

4 large collard leaves, ribs removed

FOR EACH BENTO BOX

1 c. mixed carrot and celery sticks

½ c. grapes or berries

1 oz. 70% dark chocolate

Directions

Spread 1 tablespoon hummus on every collard leaf. Divide the veggies and
chicken or tofu among the leaves and tenderly fold each up into a wrap.

Halve each wrap and present with bento box additions.

Week 2 Snack: Chocolate Avocado Pudding

Prep Time: 10 mins, Cook Time: 30 mins, Total Time: 40 mins, Serves: 4

Ingredients

2 large avocados - peeled, pitted, and cubed

1/2 cup unsweetened cocoa powder

1/2 cup brown sugar

1/3 cup coconut milk

2 teaspoons vanilla extract

1 pinch ground cinnamon

Directions

Blend avocados, cocoa powder, darker sugar, coconut milk, vanilla concentrate, and cinnamon in a blender until smooth. Refrigerate pudding until chilled, around 30 minutes.

Week 2 Dinner: Sheet-Pan Chicken Fajitas

Prep Time: 15 mins, Cook Time: 15 mins, Total Time: 30 mins, Serves: 4

Ingredients

1 tablespoon chili powder

Kosher salt and freshly ground black pepper

1 pound baby bell peppers (12 to 15 peppers), halved, stemmed and seeded

1 large yellow onion, halved and thinly sliced

2 tablespoons extra-virgin olive oil

1 1/2 pounds boneless, skinless chicken breast

Juice of 1 lime, plus lime wedges, for serving

8 fajita-size flour tortillas, warmed

Shredded Monterey Jack cheese, guacamole, hot sauce, salsa, and sour cream, for serving

Directions

Preheat the grill to high. Line a rimmed baking sheet with foil.

Mix the bean stew powder, 2 teaspoons salt, and 1 teaspoon pepper in a small bowl. Put the peppers and onions on the readied baking sheet, sprinkle with 1 tablespoon of the oil and season with a large portion of the bean stew powder mixture. Cook until soft and beginning to burn, around 10 minutes.

Meanwhile, cut the chicken into ¼-inch-thick cuts and throw in a large bowl with the rest of the chili powder mixture and 1 tablespoon oil.

After the peppers are relaxed and beginning to burn, around 10 minutes, spread the chicken over the peppers and onions and return the baking sheet to the oven until the chicken is cooked through and beginning to darken, around 5 more minutes. Sprinkle with the lime juice.

Serve with the warmed tortillas, Monterey Jack cheddar, guacamole, hot sauce, salsa, harsh cream, and lime wedges.

Week 3 Breakfast: Avocado Breakfast Bowls

Prep Time: 5 mins, Cook Time: 20 mins, Total Time: 25 mins, Serves: 4

Ingredients

1/2 cup water

1/4 cup red quinoa

1 1/2 teaspoons olive oil

2 eggs

1 pinch salt and ground black pepper to taste

1/4 teaspoon seasoned salt

1/4 teaspoon ground black pepper

1 avocado, diced

2 tablespoons crumbled feta cheese

Directions

Stir water and quinoa together in a rice cooker; cook until quinoa is delicate, around 15 minutes.

Heat olive oil in a skillet over medium heat and cook eggs to desired doneness; season with salt and pepper.

Mix quinoa and eggs in a bowl; top with avocado and feta cheddar.

Week 3 Lunch: Mediterranean Chickpea Mason Jar Salads

Prep Time: 20 mins, Cook Time: 20 mins, Total Time: 40 mins, Serves: 4

Ingredients

Red Wine Vinaigrette

1/4 cup extra-virgin olive oil

3 tablespoons red wine vinegar

2 cloves garlic, minced

1 teaspoon spicy brown mustard

1 teaspoon maple syrup

2 tablespoons water

1/2 teaspoon dried oregano

1/2 teaspoon fine sea salt

Freshly ground black pepper

Salad Assembly

1 small red onion, diced

1 English cucumber, chopped

1.5 cups cooked garbanzo beans (1 15-oz. can, drained and rinsed)

1 pint cherry tomatoes, chopped

1/2 cup crumbled feta (optional)

1 large head of romaine, chopped

Directions

Prepare the red wine vinaigrette by adding the oil, vinegar, garlic, mustard, maple syrup, water, oregano, salt, and a few drudgeries of dark pepper to a small container with a cover. (I use a small Mason container.) Shake it vivaciously to join.

Prepare 4 wide-mouth quart-sized Mason shakes on your counter for easy serving of mixed greens mixture. Pour 3 tablespoons of the dressing into the base of each one. Over the dressing, add the diced onion, cucumber, beans, cherry tomatoes, feta, and then the lettuce, in a specific order to remain separate from the spongy vegetables.

Secure the top to make the containers water/air proof and store in the fridge until ready to serve for as long as 4 days.

To serve the Mason container plate of mixed greens, unscrew the top and empty the substance into a large bowl. Since the dressing is on the base, it will pour over the salad last, dressing all of the vegetables. Mix well to coat and enjoy.

Week 3 Snack: Crunchy Keto Rosemary Crackers

Prep Time: 15 mins, Cook Time: 20 mins, Total Time: 35 mins, Serves: 4

Ingredients

1 Large whole egg

1 tablespoon olive oil

3-4 tablespoons water

1/2 teaspoon salt

1/4 teaspoon pepper

2 tablespoons rosemary

1/2 teaspoon garlic powder

1/2 cup almonds

1/2 cup pecans

1 cup pumpkin seeds

1/4 cup flax meal

Directions

Preheat oven to 325 degrees and line a large baking sheet with parchment paper. Put aside.

Whisk egg in a small bowl with water, olive oil, salt, pepper, garlic powder, and finely chopped rosemary.

Add nuts and seeds to a large food processor and blend on high until generally slashed. Add flax meal and blend to mix. Pour in fluid mixture and pulse just until blended.

Pour out mixture onto a parchment paper and take off to 1/6" thick. Cut into even pieces and transfer to the baking sheet.

Bake for 30 minutes until bright dark and soft.

Week 3 Dinner: Baked Cilantro Lime Salmon in Foil Recipe

Prep Time: 10 mins, Cook Time: 20 mins, Total Time: 30 mins, Serves: 4

Ingredients

1 lb salmon fillet, skin removed (on is ok too)

1/2 lime, juice squeezed

2 tablespoons honey

2–3 tablespoons cilantro, chopped

1–2 garlic cloves, minced

1/2 teaspoon cumin

2 tablespoons olive oil

Salt and pepper to taste

Directions

Preheat the oven to 350° Fahrenheit.

In a small bowl, mix lime juice, garlic, nectar, cilantro, olive oil, and cumin. Blend well and put aside.

Season salmon fillet with salt and pepper to taste and place on a large greased tin foil. Fold up all four sides of the foil to keep the sauce from spilling onto the counter. Pour the cilantro lime sauce over the salmon.

Fold the sides of the foil over the salmon covering completely, and seal into a closed bundle. Place lightly on oven rack and bake until cooked through, around 15-20 minutes.

Optional approach: Open the foil uncovering the tip of the salmon and cook for the last 4-5 minutes, for a sautéed top. Top with extra cilantro or lime squeeze just before serving.

Week 4 Breakfast: PB&J Overnight Oats

These PB&J Overnight Oats are loaded with smooth Peanut Butter and Chia Jam. A generous, filling, and a delicious way to enjoy the classic sandwich... for breakfast!

Prep Time: 10 mins, Cook Time: 0 mins, Total Time: 10 mins, Serves: 4

Ingredients

1 tbsp Creamy Peanut Butter

3/4 cup Filtered Water

1/2 cup Quick Cooking or Rolled Oats

1 tbsp Chia Seeds

1 tsp Maple Syrup (Optional)

2+ tbsp Chia Seed Jam

More Peanut Butter and Jam, for topping (Optional)

Directions

First, make your "Nut Milk." Add the Peanut Butter to a medium bowl and with a small amount of the Filtered Water to it. Use a rush to "mix" the PB with the fluid, and gradually stir until a smooth, Peanut Butter "Milk" shapes. Add the remainder of the Water to the bowl.

Next, add the Rolled Oats, Chia Seeds, and Maple Syrup to the bowl. Mix well and let it sit for 5 or so minutes so that the Oats can soak in the dampness.

Scoop a portion of the Oatmeal into the base of a glass container or Tupperware, and layer with Chia Seed Jam. Pour the rest of the Oatmeal on top of the Jam, and coat as you desire. I like to keep things simple with more PB and Jam!

Store in the fridge until ready to serve; the Oatmeal will stay for up to 6 days.

Week 4 Lunch: Taco Stuffed Sweet Potatoes

Prep Time: 20 mins, Cook Time: 20 mins, Total Time: 40 mins, Serves: 4

Ingredients

4 medium sweet potatoes

Olive oil

Salt and pepper

1 small onion, chopped (1/2 cup chopped)

3 garlic cloves, minced

1 pound ground beef

1/2 cup chicken broth

1 tablespoon tomato paste

2 teaspoons brown sugar

1 teaspoon salt

1 1/2 teaspoons ground chipotle (or to taste)

1 teaspoon ground coriander

1 teaspoon dried or 1/2 teaspoon ground oregano

1/2 teaspoon ground cumin

1/4 teaspoon ground cayenne

1 teaspoon cider vinegar

Shredded Mexican blend cheese

Sour cream

Avocado

Sliced green onion, for garnish

Directions

Preheat oven to 400 degrees Fahrenheit. Poke sweet potatoes all over with a fork. Rub with olive oil and sprinkle with salt and pepper. Spread on a foil-lined baking sheet and bake for 40 to 50 minutes or until fork delicate.

Meanwhile, heat 1 tablespoon olive oil in a large skillet set over medium heat. Add onion and cook until mollified and clear, 3 to 5 minutes. Add garlic and sauté until fragrant, around 30 seconds. Add hamburger and cook, separating any large pieces with the back of a spoon, for around 5 minutes or until simply cooked through. Add chicken stock, tomato paste, sugar, salt, and flavors and cook until fluid is thickened and saucy and meat is totally covered. Depending on how greasy your meat is, you might want to slowly add or reduce the chicken stock to achieve a pleasant saucy consistency. Add in vinegar.

To serve, chop a few sweet potatoes and tenderly draw open. Load up with taco filling, and top with a sprinkle of ground cheddar, avocado, acrid cream, and green onion.

Week 4 Snack: Pumpkin Pie Energy Bites

Prep Time: 20 mins, Cook Time: 0 mins, Total Time: 20 mins, Serves: 4

Ingredients

1 cup pitted dates

Warm water

½ cup raw pecan halves (or pecan pieces)

⅓ cup canned pumpkin puree

¼ cup unsweetened coconut flakes. Reserve a small amount for garnish

1 tsp. pure hazelnut extract or pure maple extract

1 tsp. pure maple syrup

2 tsp. pumpkin pie spice

1 pinch sea salt or Himalayan salt

Directions

Place dates in a medium bowl and mix with water. Let them soak for 10 minutes. Drain. Put aside.

Place pecans in food processor; blend until finely ground.

Add dates, pumpkin, coconut extract, maple syrup, pumpkin pie flavor, and salt; blend until all around mixed. Place in a medium bowl. Refrigerate for 30 minutes.

Using clean hands, fold into tablespoon-sized balls; roll in the reserved coconut flakes (if wanted).

Store refrigerated, in a closed container.

Week 4 Dinner: Chili Maple Lime Salmon Bowls with Forbidden Rice

Prep Time: 5 mins, Cook Time: 25 mins, Total Time: 30 mins, Serves: 4

Ingredients

2 (6 oz) wild salmon fillets

1 tablespoon pure maple syrup

1 small lime, juiced

1 teaspoon chili powder

3 cloves garlic, minced

1 teaspoon virgin coconut oil

1/2 cup uncooked black rice (also known as forbidden rice)

1/2 mango, diced

1/2 cup cooked shelled edamame

1/8 teaspoon salt

To garnish: Cilantro and green onion

Optional: Avocado slices

Directions

While the rice cooks, preheat oven to 400 degrees Fahrenheit. Line a large baking sheet with parchment paper to keep the coating from draining. Place salmon fillets 2 inches apart on the parchment paper, skin side down.

In a small bowl, whisk together maple syrup, lime juice, bean stew powder, and garlic. Pour or lightly brush the coating over the salmon, saving 1 tablespoon to coat the salmon once cooked. Bake for 15-20 minutes or until salmon is done and separate with a fork.

Share mango and rice mixture between two dishes, and add the salmon, topping with green onion and cilantro if desired.

If you time this effectively, this can easily be a 30-minute meal all the way.

Week 5 Breakfast: loaded breakfast stuffed peppers

Prep Time: 10 mins, Cook Time: 25 mins, Total Time: 35 mins, Serves: 4

Ingredients

4 large bell peppers, whatever color you like

9 large eggs

1/2 cup fully cooked breakfast potatoes*

1/2 cup cooked quinoa

1/2 cup black beans

1/2 cup chopped spinach leaves

1/3 cup shredded cheese, plus more for topping if desired

1 teaspoon salt

1/4 teaspoon black pepper

Directions

Pre-heat the oven to 400 degrees Fahrenheit. Cut the peppers down the middle and remove the seeds. You can either slice them down the middle width-wise or length-wise but they will most likely hold better if you cut them width-wise. Place the peppers on a baking sheet and bake for 5 minutes.

Crack the eggs into a large mixing bowl and beat with a fork. Add the rest of the ingredients and mix until combined.

Remove the peppers from the oven and spoon the egg mixture into each pepper, depending on how huge your peppers are. Sprinkle the top of each pepper with cheddar and place back in the oven and bake peppers until eggs are set, around 20 minutes. Serve eggs quickly and top with chopped herbs if desired.

Week 5 Lunch: Steak Cobb Salad Meal Prep

Lime juice and cilantro are the key ingredients to making this delicious, healthy salad you'll want to make all spring. Made with cooked stripped shrimp and the freshest ingredients – avocados, tomatoes, red onion, cilantro and hacked jalapeño hurled with some crisply crushed lime juice and a pinch of olive oil.

Prep Time: 25 mins, Cook Time: 15 mins, Total Time: 40 mins, Serves: 4

Ingredients

- 2 tablespoons unsalted butter
- 1 pound steak
- 2 tablespoons olive oil
- Kosher salt and freshly ground black pepper, to taste
- 6 large eggs
- 6 cups baby spinach
- 1 cup cherry tomatoes, halved
- 1 cup Fisher Nuts Pecan Halves
- 1/2 cup crumbled feta cheese

Directions

Melt butter in a large skillet over medium-high heat.

Using paper towels, pat the two sides of the steak dry. Sprinkle with olive oil; season with salt and pepper, to taste.

Add steak to the skillet and cook, flipping once, until cooked through to wanted doneness, around 3-4 minutes for every side for medium-rare. Let the meat cool before dicing into small pieces.

Place eggs in a large pan and cover with cold water about 1 inch. Heat to the point of boiling and cook for 1 minute. Spread eggs with a tight-fitting lid and reduce from heat; set aside for 8-10 minutes. Drain well and let cool before peeling and dicing.

To prepare the salad, place spinach into meal prep containers; top with pieces of steak, eggs, tomatoes, pecans, and feta.

Serve with balsamic vinaigrette, or desired dressing.

Week 5 Snack: Banana Bread Baked Oatmeal With Berries And Cinnamon

Prep Time: 20 mins, Cook Time: 20 mins, Total Time: 40 mins, Serves: 4

Ingredients

2 1/4 cups old fashioned rolled oats

1 teaspoon baking powder

1 teaspoon ground cinnamon

1/4 teaspoon salt

1 cup ripe mashed bananas, about 2 large bananas or 3 medium bananas

3/4 cup almond milk

1 large egg

1 teaspoon vanilla extract

1/2 cup blueberries, fresh or frozen

1/2 cup sliced strawberries, fresh or frozen

1/2 cup raspberries, fresh or frozen

Directions

Preheat oven to 350 degrees. Grease an 8x8 square baking pan (or another medium baking pan) with coconut oil or cooking splash and set aside.

In a large mixing bowl, mix together the oats, preparing powder, cinnamon, and salt. Set aside.

In another mixing bowl, whisk together the mashed banana, almond milk, egg, and vanilla extract. Add the wet ingredients to the dry ingredients and mix until everything is combined.

Add in the blueberries, strawberries, and raspberries and empty the oat mixture into the baking pan.

Bake for 35 to 40 minutes or until the top is set and dark brown.

Remove from the oven and allow to cool for 10 to 15 minutes. Slice and serve warm, or completely cool, cover tightly and refrigerate until ready to enjoy.

Week 5 Dinner: Vegetarian Tofu Cashew Coconut Curry

Prep Time: 20 mins, Cook Time: 20 mins, Total Time: 40 mins, Serves: 4

Ingredients

- 1 tablespoon virgin coconut oil
- 3 cloves garlic, minced
- 1 tablespoon freshly grated ginger
- 1 jalapeño, diced
- 1 medium sweet potato, diced into 1-inch cubes
- ½ head of cauliflower, cut into small florets (about 2-3 cups)
- 1 bell yellow or orange pepper, diced
- 2 carrots, thinly diced or chopped
- 2 tablespoons curry powder
- ½ teaspoon turmeric
- ½ teaspoon cumin
- ⅛ teaspoon ground cinnamon
- ½ teaspoon salt

1 (15 oz) can lite coconut milk

1/2 cup tomato sauce

½ cup vegetarian broth

¼ cup roasted cashews, ground

1 package firm or extra firm Nasoya tofu, drained and cubed

To garnish: Cilantro and extra cashews

Directions

Add coconut oil to a large pot and spot over medium-high heat. Add garlic, ginger, jalapeno, sweet potato, cauliflower, bell pepper, and carrots. Saute for 10 minutes, mixing frequently, until carrots begin to soften.

Next, mix in curry powder, turmeric, cumin, cinnamon, and salt. Add coconut milk, tomato sauce, vegan soup and ground cashews. Stir until smooth. Gently add tofu and mix. Cook on low heat for 20 minutes or until sweet potatoes and carrots are fork tender. Serve immediately with cilantro.

Week 6 Breakfast: Instant Pot Cinnamon Roll French Toast Casserole

Prep Time: 15 mins, Cook Time: 25 mins, Total Time: 40 mins, Serves: 4

Ingredients

French Toast

1 loaf (12 slices) sourdough bread, sliced into 1-inch cubes (~6 cups)

8 large eggs

1 cup milk, any kind

1 teaspoon vanilla extract

2 tablespoons maple syrup

1/2 cup walnuts, chopped

Almond Butter Cinnamon Drizzle

2/3 cup almond butter, drippy

2 tablespoons maple syrup

3 teaspoons ground cinnamon

1 tablespoon melted coconut oil*

Optional Topping

4 tablespoons butter, chilled

1/4 cup brown sugar

Directions

Spray a 7 – 8-inch glass bowl with coconut oil cooking spray. This is the bowl you will use to cook your French toast in. Set aside.

Next, in a small bowl mix together all the ingredients for the almond butter cinnamon drizzle. The consistency ought to be drippy and if it's not, add extra melted coconut oil.

In a medium bowl, whisk eggs, milk, vanilla, and maple syrup.

Place some of the bread cubes and half of the walnuts into the glass bowl. Drizzle on half of the almond butter cinnamon drizzle over the bread mixture. Add the rest of the bread cubes and drizzle on the remaining walnuts and cinnamon drizzle over the bread.

Pour egg mixture over the whole thing and mix bread cubes with the egg mixture using a spatula. Then, sprinkle on the optional topping.

Place metal Instant Pot trivet on the bottom of Instant Pot and pour in some water. Then, place French toast bowl over the trivet.

Lock Instant Pot and turn pressure valve to seal. Press manual and turn to high pressure and cook for 25 minutes.

Quick release and remove Instant Pot cover. Let cool and then serve with maple syrup.

Week 6 Lunch: Creamy Vegan Mexican Pasta Salad

Prep Time: 15 mins, Cook Time: 15 mins, Total Time: 30 mins, Serves: 4

Ingredients

10 ounces whole-wheat or gluten-free pasta

5 slices Sweet Earth Natural Foods Benevolent Bacon

1/2 cup raw cashews, soaked in water overnight or at least 4 hours*

1/2 cup salsa

1/2 cup unsweetened non-dairy milk

2 garlic cloves (1 teaspoon minced)

1 teaspoon chilli powder

3/4 teaspoon cumin

1/2 teaspoon smoked paprika

Salt and pepper, to taste

1/2 cup black beans, drained and rinsed

1/2 cup corn (defrosted if frozen)

1 large bell pepper, diced

Fresh cilantro, for garnish

Directions

Cook pasta as indicated on the package. Drain.

In a skillet or cast iron pan, grease lightly with oil. Over medium heat, add 5 slices of Benevolent Bacon. Cook for 2-3 minutes, then flip. Remove from heat. When cool, slice into small pieces. Set aside.

To a blender or food processor, add cashews, salsa, milk, garlic, chilli powder, cumin, and paprika. Blend until smooth; season with salt and pepper, if needed.

In a large bowl, add pasta, black beans, corn, bell pepper, and bacon pieces. Pour the cashews dressing on top; mix to combine until all ingredients are mixed.

Week 6 Snack: Parmesan Roasted Snap Peas

Prep Time: 10 mins, Cook Time: 2 mins, Total Time: 12 mins, Serves: 4

Ingredients

8 oz Mann's Stringless Sugar Snap Peas

2 teaspoons olive oil

1/4 cup panko breadcrumbs

1/2 cup parmesan cheese

1 teaspoon lemon zest

Directions

Heat oven to 425°F. Line a baking sheet with parchment paper and set aside.

Toss the peas with olive oil, salt, and pepper, then with the parmesan, panko breadcrumbs, and lemon pizzazz.

Spread on the baking sheet and bake in the oven for 8-10 minutes.

Serve immediately.

Week 6 Dinner: Cheesy Chicken Quinoa Enchilada Meatloaf Muffins

Prep Time: 20 mins, Cook Time: 20 mins, Total Time: 40 mins, Serves: 4

Ingredients

For the quinoa:

1/3 cup uncooked quinoa

2/3 cup water

For the muffins:

4 cloves of garlic

1/2 cup finely chopped yellow onion

1 red or orange pepper, finely diced

1 teaspoon olive oil

1 teaspoon cumin

1 teaspoon dried oregano

1 teaspoon chili powder

A few dashes of your favorite hot sauce

A few dashes red pepper flakes, if desired

1/2 cup chopped cilantro

Freshly ground salt and black pepper, to taste

3/4 cup red enchilada sauce, divided

1 pound ground chicken or lean ground turkey breast

2 egg whites (or 1 egg)

2/3 cup reduced fat shredded colby jack or mexican cheese

Directions

To cook quinoa: In a small pot, heat water and quinoa to a boil. Cover, reduce heat to low and let simmer for 15 minutes or until quinoa has absorbed all of the liquid. Remove from heat and separate quinoa with fork; set aside to cool for 5 minutes. While the quinoa cooks you can proceed to the next stage.

Preheat oven to 350 degrees F. Spray a 12-container biscuit tin generously with olive oil. Heat olive oil in a medium skillet over medium heat. Add garlic, onion, and bell pepper. Cook for a few minutes or until the onions soften. Transfer to a large bowl to cool for several minutes.

Add cooked quinoa, cumin, oregano, chili powder, hot sauce, red pepper flakes, cilantro, salt and pepper and half of the enchilada sauce (reserve the rest to top the muffins later). Next, mix in ground chicken (or turkey) and egg whites and 1/4 amount of the cheddar. You may need to use your hands to ensure all the ingredients around together. Use a 1/4 container measuring glass or a frozen yogurt scoop to add meatloaf mixture equally to the muffin cups.

Bake for 25-30 minutes. Remove from oven and spoon the remaining enchilada sauce and cheddar over the top of the muffins. Place back in the oven and bake for an extra 3-5 minutes or until the cheese melts and muffins are cooked. Let cool for a few minutes, then serve with fresh vegetables for a full meal.

Chapter 21: Freezer Meals

Crockpot Vegetarian Garden Vegetable Soup with Pesto (Panera Copycat)

Prep Time: 20 mins, Cook Time: 20 mins, Total Time: 40 mins, Serves: 4

Ingredients

2 cans of diced tomatoes (14.5oz each), undrained

1 small zucchini, diced

1/2lb fresh green beans, ends cut off and chopped

2.5oz fresh baby spinach (about 3 big handfuls)

1 small yellow onion, peeled and diced (1 cup)

1 small red bell pepper, diced

1/4-1/2 cup pearled barley (not quick cooking)

4 cloves garlic, minced

2 tablespoons honey

1 tablespoon brown sugar

2 tablespoons Italian seasonings

1 bay leaf

4 cups vegetable broth *not needed until day of cooking

6 tablespoons pesto (store-bought or homemade) *not needed until day of cooking

Directions

Add all ingredients to your crockpot (except pesto).

Cook on "low" setting for 8 hours or until vegetables are soft.

Remove bay leaf.

Scoop into bowls and top with pesto.

To Freeze and Cook Later

Label a gallon-sized plastic fridge pack with the name of the recipe, use-by date (3 months from the prep date), and cooking instructions.

To your freezer bag, add all ingredients except broth and pesto.

Remove as much air as possible, seal, and freeze for up to three months.

When ready to eat, defrost for some time in the fridge or in the morning in water.

Add to crockpot with broth and cook for 8 hours on "low."

Remove bay leaf and serve into bowls with pesto.

Crockpot Chicken Soup with Mexican Seasonings

Cook crisp or freeze to cook later. We love eating our soup with shredded cheddar and tortilla chips.

Prep Time: 20 mins, Cook Time: 20 mins, Total Time: 40 mins, Serves: 4

Ingredients

- 1 pound carrots, peeled and diced
- 1 medium-sized yellow onion, diced
- 2 large cloves of garlic, minced
- 2 roma tomatoes, chopped

1 cup tomato juice (If you buy a big can/bottle, freeze the extra in ice cubes trays for future soups and chili's)

1 teaspoons cumin

1 teaspoon fennel seeds

1 teaspoons chili powder

1 teaspoon salt

Juice from 1/2 lime (about 2 tablespoons)

1 pound boneless skinless chicken breasts

4 cups fat-free, reduced-sodium chicken broth (If freezing, this is not needed until day of cooking)

Directions

Mix all ingredients in crockpot and cook for 4-8 hours, or until carrots are soft and chicken is cooked through.

Shred chicken with a fork and mix.

TO FREEZE AND COOK LATER

Mix all ingredients (except chicken broth) in a gallon-sized plastic freezer bag. Remove as much air as possible and freeze for up to three months.

To cook, defrost and add to crockpot with chicken broth. Cook on "low" setting for 4-8 hours, or until carrots are soft and chicken is cooked through. Shred chicken with a fork and stir.

Freezer Meal Wild Rice Soup

Prep Time: 15 mins, Cook Time: 25 mins, Total Time: 40 mins, Serves: 4

Ingredients

3 cups mirepoix, fresh or frozen

8 ounces mushrooms, fresh or frozen

3 cloves garlic, minced

1 cup uncooked wild rice (the REAL stuff, not a blend)

4 cups vegetable or chicken broth

1 teaspoon salt

1 teaspoon poultry seasoning (or spices like sage, thyme, and rosemary)

1 lb. chicken breasts (optional)

ADD AFTER COOKING:

6 tablespoons butter

1/2 cup flour

1 1/2 cups whole milk

Directions

INSTANT POT: From frozen, 30 minutes on high pressure + 10 minutes normal release.

SLOW COOKER: From frozen, 4 hours on high.

Last STEP: Melt butter, add in flour, whisk in milk until rich and thick. Add to the soup. Add extra water to thin to desired consistency.

Slow Cooker Sausage Spinach Tomato Soup Recipe

Prep Time: 20 mins, Cook Time: 20 mins, Total Time: 40 mins, Serves: 4

Ingredients

1 lb ground sweet or spicy Italian sausage (We prefer spicy. Note: If you can only find sausage links, remove the casing before cooking.)

24 oz jar of pasta sauce

1 can of cannellini beans, drained and rinsed

1 box of frozen chopped spinach

1/2 pound of carrots (about 4 large carrots), peeled and chopped into bite-sized pieces

1 small yellow onion, diced (about one cup)

4 cups of chicken broth

1 cup uncooked pasta (I like to use elbow macaroni or ditalini)

Directions

Brown the sausage in a pan.

Add the sausage and the rest of the ingredients (except the pasta) to your slow cooker and cook on the "low" setting for 6-8 hours.

Add pasta the last 15 minutes of cooking and turn the heat to "high."

To Freeze and Cook Later

Add all ingredients to a gallon-sized plastic freezer bag (except chicken broth and pasta). When ready to eat, defrost for some time in the fridge and throw into your slow cooker with chicken soup. Cook on "low" setting for 6-8 hours or until the sausage is cooked through. Add pasta and turn the heat to "high."

Serve with garlic bread.

Freezer Meal Soup Recipes | Vegetable Beef Soup

This delicious Vegetable Beef Soup is one of my favorite fridge meal soup recipes. Ideal all year round, easy to freeze, and quick to warm – it's sure to please!

Prep Time: 20 mins, Cook Time: 20 mins, Total Time: 40 mins, Serves: 4

Ingredients

> 4 lbs lean ground beef cooked with one diced onion and 5 diced celery stalks
>
> 80 oz frozen Peas, Carrots, Corn (I buy Birds Eye Mixed Vegetables, 5 lb bag at Walmart)
>
> 4 29-oz cans of Crushed tomatoes
>
> 6 qts broth (I used chicken broth because it's what I had on hand, but you can also use beef)
>
> 1 tbs dill weed
>
> Salt/Pepper per taste preference

Directions

> In a large pan, cook 4 lbs of lean ground beef with one diced onion and 5 diced

celery stalks until completely cooked. Break and drain.

In a large stock pot, mix 4 lbs of cooked and drained ground beef, 6 quarts broth, 4 29-oz jars of crushed tomatoes, 1 tbs dill weed, and 80 oz sack on frozen peas, corn, carrots. Simmer on medium heat stirring gently as needed.

Freezer Meal Soup Directions

Once soup is safely cooled, scoop into freezer safe soup containers. Leave room for soup to expand during freezing. Here is my Amazon member interface for the fridge soup compartments I used this go round.

Store soup for up to 3-months in the refrigerator.

For use, simply set out into the fridge the night before or morning before needed. Warm the soup in the microwave or on the stove top when needed. I've even warmed my freezer meal soup recipes in the slow cooker on low heat for up to two hours.

Serve as a full meal or with fresh salad and a sandwich!

Chapter 22: Shopping Lists

1st week Shopping list

- 21 Pieces eggs
- 28 grams coconut flour
- 50 grams granulated sweetener
- 4 grams baking powder
- 9 grams vanilla
- 45 grams full fat milk or cream
- 125 grams butter melted
- 60 grams red onion
- 4 green onion total within 40 grams
- 2 limes
- 4.57 grams olive oil
- 5 grams Salt
- 5 grams Flaky sea salt
- 1grams black pepper
- 453.6 grams shrimp
- 1 medium tomato
- 8 grape
- 1 medium Hass avocado
- 1 jalapeno
- 1 gram cilantro
- 360 grams dark chocolate chips
- 30 grams vegetable oil
- 60 grams salted pretzels
- 60 grams dried cherries
- 60 grams unsweetened coconut flakes

- 60 grams unsalted pistachios
- 150 grams shiitake mushrooms
- 140 grams shredded napa cabbage
- 3.5 grams peeled grated ginger root
- 2 cloves garlic, minced
- 10 grams white or yellow miso (soybean paste)
- 10 grams reduced sodium soy sauce
- 150 grams Swanson® Certified Organic Vegetable Broth or Swanson® Vegetable Broth
- 300 grams spiralized zucchini noodles (about 14 ounces)
- 50 grams shredded red cabbage
- 50 grams fresh spinach, roughly chopped
- 50 grams shredded mozzarella cheese

2nd week Shopping list

- 60 grams hummus
- 1 medium cucumber, peeled and sliced into matchsticks
- 2 medium carrots, peeled and sliced into matchsticks
- 1 c. shredded purple cabbage
- 2 avocados, pitted and sliced
- 3 oz. shredded chicken or sautéed tofu
- 4 large collard leaves
- 1 c. mixed carrot and celery sticks

- 100 grams grapes or berries
- 1 oz. 70% dark chocolate
- 2 large avocados - peeled, pitted, and cubed
- 50 grams unsweetened cocoa powder
- 50 grams brown sugar
- 75 grams coconut milk
- 20 grams vanilla extract
- 1 pinch ground cinnamon
- 15 grams chili powder
- Kosher salt and freshly ground black pepper
- 1 pound baby bell peppers (12 to 15 peppers), halved, stemmed and seeded
- 1 large yellow onion, halved and thinly sliced
- 15 grams extra-virgin olive oil
- 1 1/2 pounds boneless, skinless chicken breast
- Juice of 1 lime, plus lime wedges, for serving
- 8 fajita-size flour tortillas, warmed
- Shredded Monterey Jack cheese, guacamole, hot sauce, salsa and sour cream

3rd week Shopping list

- 150 ml water
- 50 grams red quinoa

- 50 grams olive oil
- 2 eggs
- 1 pinch salt and ground black pepper to taste
- 50 grams seasoned salt
- 50 grams ground black pepper
- 1 avocado, diced
- 50 grams crumbled feta cheese
- 150 grams extra-virgin olive oil
- 60 grams red wine vinegar
- 2 cloves garlic , minced
- 100 grams spicy brown mustard
- 50 grams maple syrup
- 50 grams dried oregano
- 50 grams fine sea salt
- 1 small red onion
- 1 English cucumber
- 1 15-oz cooked garbanzo beans
- 1 pint cherry tomatoes
- 1 large head of romaine
- 1 Large whole egg
- 50 grams olive oil
- 50 grams salt
- 20 grams pepper
- 70 grams rosemary
- 100 grams garlic powder
- 150 grams almonds
- 100 grams pecans
- 200 grams pumpkin seeds

- ➢ 50 grams flax meal
- ➢ 1 lb salmon filet, skin removed
- ➢ 1/2 lime, juice squeezed
- ➢ 20 grams honey
- ➢ 30 grams cilantro
- ➢ 1–2 garlic cloves
- ➢ 40 grams cumin
- ➢ 60 grams olive oil

4th Week Shopping list

- ➢ 1 tbsp Creamy Peanut Butter
- ➢ 3/4 cup Filtered Water
- ➢ 1/2 cup Quick Cooking
- ➢ 1 tbsp Chia Seeds
- ➢ 1 tsp Maple Syrup
- ➢ 2+ tbsp Chia Seed Jam
- ➢ More Peanut Butter and Jam, for topping
- ➢ 4 medium sweet potatoes
- ➢ olive oil
- ➢ salt and pepper
- ➢ 1 small onion
- ➢ 3 garlic cloves
- ➢ 1 pound ground beef
- ➢ 1/2 cup chicken broth
- ➢ 1 tablespoon tomato paste
- ➢ 2 teaspoons brown sugar
- ➢ 1 teaspoon salt
- ➢ 1 1/2 teaspoons ground chipotle

- 1 teaspoon ground coriander
- 1 teaspoon dried or 1/2 teaspoon ground oregano
- 1/2 teaspoon ground cumin
- 1/4 teaspoon ground cayenne
- 1 teaspoon cider vinegar
- shredded Mexican blend cheese
- sour cream
- avocado
- sliced green onion, for garnish
- 1 cup pitted dates
- Warm water
- ½ cup raw pecan halves
- ⅓ cup canned pumpkin puree
- ¼ cup unsweetened coconut flakes reserve small amount for garnish
- 1 tsp. pure hazelnut extract or pure maple extract
- 1 tsp. pure maple syrup
- 2 tsp. pumpkin pie spice
- 1 pinch sea salt or Himalayan salt
- 2 (6 oz) wild salmon filets
- 1 tablespoon pure maple syrup
- 1 small lime, juiced
- 1 teaspoon chili powder
- 3 cloves garlic, minced
- 1 teaspoon virgin coconut oil
- 1/2 cup uncooked black rice
- 1/2 mango, diced

- 1/2 cup cooked shelled edamame
- 1/8 teaspoon salt

5th Week shopping list

- 4 large bell peppers
- 9 large eggs
- 1/2 cup fully cooked breakfast potato
- 1/2 cup cooked quinoa
- 1/2 cup black beans
- 1/2 cup chopped spinach leaves
- 1/3 cup shredded cheese, plus more for topping if desired
- 1 teaspoon salt
- 1/4 teaspoon black pepper
- 2 tablespoons unsalted butter
- 1 pound steak
- 2 tablespoons olive oil
- Kosher salt and freshly ground black pepper, to taste
- 6 large eggs
- 6 cups baby spinach
- 1 cup cherry tomatoes, halved
- 1 cup Fisher Nuts Pecan Halves
- 1/2 cup crumbled feta cheese
- 2 1/4 cups old fashioned rolled oats
- 1 teaspoon baking powder
- 1 teaspoon ground cinnamon
- 1/4 teaspoon salt

- 1 cup ripe mashed bananas, about 2 large bananas or 3 medium bananas
- 3/4 cup almond milk
- 1 large egg
- 1 teaspoon vanilla extract
- 1/2 cup blueberries, fresh or frozen
- 1/2 cup sliced strawberries, fresh or frozen
- 1/2 cup raspberries, fresh or frozen
- 1 tablespoon virgin coconut oil
- 3 cloves garlic, minced
- 1 tablespoon freshly grated ginger
- 1 jalapeño, diced
- 1 medium sweet potato, diced into 1 inch cubes
- ½ head of cauliflower, cut into small florets
- 1 bell yellow or orange pepper
- 2 carrots, thinly diced or chopped
- 2 tablespoons curry powder
- ½ teaspoon turmeric
- ½ teaspoon cumin
- ⅛ teaspoon ground cinnamon
- ½ teaspoon salt
- 1 (15 oz) can lite coconut milk
- 1/2 cup tomato sauce
- ½ cup vegetarian broth
- ¼ cup roasted cashews

- 1 package firm or extra firm Nasoya tofu, drained and cubed
- To garnish: Cilantro and extra cashews

6th Week shopping list

- 10 large eggs
- 1 cup milk
- 1 teaspoon vanilla extract
- 2 tablespoons maple syrup
- 1/2 cups walnuts, chopped
- 2/3 cup almond butter, drippy
- 2 tablespoons maple syrup
- 3 teaspoons ground cinnamon
- 1 tablespoon melted coconut oil
- 4 tablespoons butter
- 50 grams brown sugar
- 10 ounces whole-wheat or gluten-free pasta
- 5 slices Sweet Earth Natural Foods Benevolent Bacon
- 1/2 cup raw cashews, soaked in water overnight or at least 4 hours
- 1/2 cup salsa
- 1/2 cup unsweetened non-dairy milk
- 2 garlic cloves
- 1 teaspoon chili powder
- 3/4 teaspoon cumin
- 1/2 teaspoon smoked paprika
- Salt and pepper, to taste

- 1/2 cup black beans, drained and rinsed
- 1/2 cup corn
- 1 large bell pepper
- Fresh cilantro, for garnish
- 8 oz Mann's Stringless Sugar Snap Peas
- 2 teaspoons olive oil
- 1/4 cup panko breadcrumbs
- 1/2 cup parmesan cheese
- 1 teaspoon lemon zest
- 1/3 cup uncooked quinoa
- 2/3 cup water
- 4 cloves of garlic
- 1/2 cup finely chopped yellow onion
- 1 red or orange pepper
- 1 teaspoon olive oil
- 1 teaspoon cumin
- 1 teaspoon dried oregano
- 1 teaspoon chili powder
- few dashes of your favorite hot sauce
- few dashes red pepper flakes, if desired
- 1/2 cup chopped cilantro
- freshly ground salt and black pepper, to taste
- 3/4 cup red enchilada sauce
- 1 pound ground chicken or lean ground turkey breast
- 2/3 cup reduced fat shredded colby jack

www.ingramcontent.com/pod-product-compliance
Lightning Source LLC
Chambersburg PA
CBHW051544020426
42333CB00016B/2096